A Women's Health Survival Guide

HELPING YOU BECOME YOUR BEST SELF

Cheryl Agranovich, RN, BSN, MPH

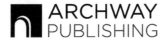 ARCHWAY PUBLISHING

Archway Publishing books may be ordered
through booksellers or by contacting:

Archway Publishing
1663 Liberty Drive
Bloomington, IN 47403
www.archwaypublishing.com
1 (888) 242-5904

ISBN: 978-1-4808-9400-6 (sc)
ISBN: 978-1-4808-9402-0 (hc)
ISBN: 978-1-4808-9401-3 (e)

Library of Congress Control Number: 2020914806

Print information available on the last page.

Archway Publishing rev. date: 06/17/2021

This book is dedicated in loving memory to
Dina Agranovich, who will live forever in our hearts.
Thank you for being our guardian angel.

Contents

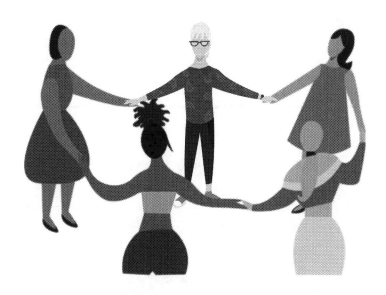

Preface

$\mathcal{I}$ created this guide not only as a practitioner but also as a patient, a survivor, and a woman who has experienced the American health-care system from both sides of the examination table. Throughout my childhood, I was pretty much on my own emotionally and financially independent since the age of seventeen. Somehow, I always knew that education would be my way forward, but it was difficult for me to complete my schooling, given that I had no financial support and was still dealing with the wounds from my childhood. At twenty-one years old and at the lowest point in my life, I had two choices: live or die. It took me weeks of serious contemplation, but I chose to get help. There is a whole other story in that journey, and I will not take your time now because we need to focus on you. Anyway, that was the point in my life when I made the promise to care about myself in the loving and kind way that I cared for others. Thankfully, with treatment, I was ultimately able to overcome my personal and deeply challenging health issues. **That was a turning point in my life for me.** I felt extremely lucky to have been given a second chance in life, and for this reason, I have focused my entire career on helping others live healthier and happier lives as well.

Early in my career, I worked as a registered nurse in an emergency room, where my interest quickly shifted toward preventive health care and corporate health management. The reason for the change of heart was because I saw way too many people who could have avoided the emergency room if they'd only thought about preventive health sooner: the diabetics with uncontrolled sugar levels, the heart attacks that could have been avoided, the parents not properly dispensing asthma medication for their children to avoid asthma attacks, and the multiple driving fatalities because people did not wear seat belts or helmets.

Over the next twenty years, I combined my passion for prevention and love for entrepreneurship to successfully build and sell two health-related companies. For me, the best parts of this experience were working in our family-friendly environment with an amazing team, helping to influence millions of people's lifestyles positively, and the fabulous clients we got to work with. Some of our clients included Mars Incorporated, Nestle, Bristol Myers Squibb, Nationwide, Parker, Eaton Corporation, HARMAN International, Campbell Soup Company, and IKEA.

However, after three decades in the health-care industry and as a working mother who was committed to balancing life at work and home, the inadequacy of the health resources we provided for women only became more obvious to me. I have watched women struggle to find the time to get the prenatal care, preventive medicine, and reproductive care they needed to live their healthiest lives amid substandard health insurance access and the inherent inequality of America's gender norms. I have witnessed so many women only taking time off from work to care for their children's or parents' health needs and putting their own health last on their list.

Over the years, I have also seen time and again what I had learned from my personal experience with healing: even though every element of a woman's health is connected, from physical to mental to sexual and even financial, women were not receiving the effective guidance needed on those topics in particular. That is why I wanted to focus this book on women specifically.

My life experiences up to this point have strengthened my resolve that we can and must do better to take care of our health. For that reason, I am now focusing on philanthropic efforts in health care full-time. **Please note that all proceeds from this book and any speaking engagements will be used to fund scholarships for young women in need to get their formal health education and to support other women's health issues.** I hope that this workbook can help change your life for the better—the way my life was changed all those years ago.

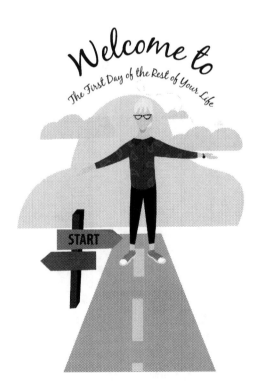

Welcome to
The First Day of the Rest of Your Life

START

Why Make Your Health a Priority?

*T*he point of this guide is to provide women with the tools they need to prioritize their own health every day, which will ultimately enable them to better achieve *all* their goals.

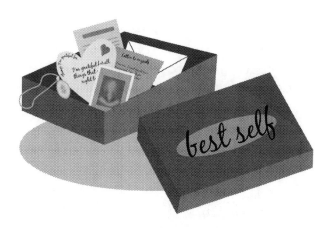

As women, we are told to juggle many things, from work to family to unrealistic body image expectations, but what no one seems to tell us to do is prioritize our own health. We are told, at a minimum, to have a few screenings once we get to certain ages and to check our breasts in the shower for lumps. Taking breast health as one example, it seems that just checking your breasts to make sure you don't already

WHY MAKE YOUR HEALTH A PRIORITY?

have breast cancer is an insane, outdated, and reactive approach to our health. What about screenings, family history, and guidance from your gynecologist?

In the twenty-first century, so much is known about long-term health, but we don't seem to talk about it, much less apply it! That's why in this guide I have broken it down into digestible, comprehensive parts to make it easy for you to use. I know what you're likely thinking: I don't have any spare time! However, you have to understand that it will require a shift in priorities to put your health at the top of your consideration set. Just remember that it's literally the only way to give yourself a longer and healthier life. There really is no more important priority than that, for your health contributes to and enables all of your other goals and priorities.

It's as simple as this: as women, we seem to have the time— or make the time—to take care of everyone else but ourselves. But if we don't start taking care of ourselves, we won't be around to keep taking care of others. Let me say that again: If we don't start taking care of ourselves, we won't be around to keep taking care of others. What I am suggesting is that you must choose to treat your body as if it is someone you love before it is too late and you have a lifestyle-related health condition that sickens or kills you.

Don't just take it from me. Here are the facts you need to know:

1. Research shows your current health is greatly affected by lifestyle-related issues and that less than 3 percent of Americans are living a healthy life.[1]

2. Six out of ten Americans have a chronic health condition, many caused by lifestyle choices such as

smoking, overuse of alcohol, poor diet, lack of physical activity, and inadequate relief of ongoing stress.[2]

3. An estimated 30.3 million people in the United States, or 9.4 percent of the population, have diabetes. About one in four people with diabetes doesn't know they have the disease. Having diabetes greatly increases a person's risk of developing heart disease, nerve damage, eye problems, and kidney disease.[3]

4. One in eight women will develop breast cancer in her lifetime.[4]

5. Based on BMI, about two out of three American women are considered overweight or obese.[5]

But it's not too late! Did you know that the progression of many lifestyle diseases can be halted if caught early enough or simply by making healthier lifestyle choices? Let's look at heart disease, which happens to be the leading cause of death in women.[6] According to the Preventive Medicine Research Institute, heart disease is reversible.[7] To reverse the downward spiral requires changing behavior and improving your lifestyle, but given the right conditions, the body has the miraculous ability to heal itself.[8] **No matter where you are in your journey to good health, today is the first day of the rest of your life.** It is never too late to start taking better care of yourself, regardless of your age or current health. It is true that aging impacts our health and lifestyle, but taking care of yourself today can improve your quality of life and even slow down the aging process. When a body is young, it can ride the crest of youth and avoid feeling the immediate effects of current lifestyle choices. This invincible nature makes it difficult to see the "future you." However, the choices you make daily, even if you are in your twenties or thirties, can affect the kind of life you have in your forties, fifties, sixties, and beyond. Just changing simple things—such as how you eat and making sure you get enough exercise and sleep— can have a dramatic impact!

Good Health Doesn't Just Happen

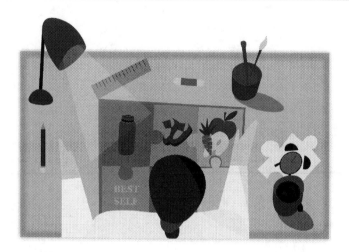

Unfortunately, you can't just wave a magic wand to make yourself healthy. It will require a considerable commitment on your part. It starts with loving yourself enough to prompt you to take better care of you. **I believe that if you can commit to loving yourself (as if it is somebody you love), you will be able to make some magical improvements.**

The hardest part about changing our lives seems to be finding the time. When I was caring for my family and working full-time, finding the time to change my health habits was difficult. Here are some practical things to keep in mind as you start to make your health a priority:

1. Identify *why* you want to change. Are you doing it for yourself, your family, or for some other reason? You might just want to feel better each day, have

more energy, or improve your current health risks. It is important to figure this out, for your reasons for change will be the foundation of your success and will continue to motivate you.

2. Recognize that change is a process of relearning and developing new habits, and enjoy that process; don't just focus on the outcome or the goal. Small steps that you will make should be celebrated too.

3. Surround yourself with people who will lift you up and support these new goals. This can be tough because as you go through this process, you may have to reevaluate your key relationships to ensure that you have a supportive team surrounding you, providing support and encouragement.

Getting Started with This Guide

As you read, you will notice that each section contains four parts:

1. **Brief Topic Intro:** I will share some of my personal anecdotes, some of my friend/client experiences, and general thoughts on why this topic is worth prioritizing.

2. **Facts You Need to Know:** I feel that these points will help you truly think about the importance and impact of the topic. I will share some important facts and statistics for you to consider as you think about your current health and additional reasons for wanting to improve your lifestyle choices.

3. **Essential Info:** In this part, you will learn about the topic and be provided with practical, easy, and effective ways to make lifestyle/health improvements. In these sections—*Creating Your Health Team, Being Your Own Health Warrior, Focusing on Nutrition, Maintaining Sustainable Fitness, Getting Enough Sleep, Prioritizing Your Mental Health, Finding Your Passion, Paying Attention to Your Sexual Health, and Navigating Your Financial Health*—you will have the chance to utilize worksheets to start creating your own personal health plan.

4. **Take Charge of Your Health:** To put your learning into action, I will provide suggestions for easy things you can start doing right away to take charge after reading so that you can incorporate your new knowledge into your life.

I wanted to make this guide easy to use, and there is some logic to the layout. The guide starts with helping you understand why you want to make your health a priority and then moves into building a foundation of good health. This foundation includes guidelines to help you create your health team and learn how to take charge of your health by being your health warrior. Next you will learn practical and effective ways to improve your daily health habits; this section targets hydration, nutrition, fitness, and sleep. Following daily health habits, mental and emotional health is also addressed and will support you as you think about prioritizing your mental health, find your passions in life, and attend to your sexual health needs. Finally, guidance on how to navigate your financial health will round out the guide.

Good luck—and congratulations on starting this new, healthier phase of your life!

Building the Foundation

$\mathcal{B}$uilding your solid health foundation starts with two key components—a supportive and comprehensive health team and you acting as your health warrior. In the next two parts, you will learn about these essential elements as well as how they can form your solid health foundation.

CREATING YOUR HEALTH TEAM

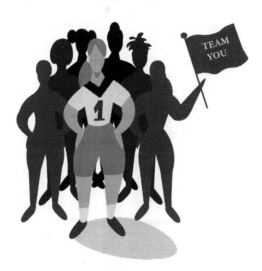

To project the importance of creating your own health team, I want to start by sharing a client story from when I was managing my health promotion practice. The employee was a thirty-eight-year-old single mom who participated in an on-site health screening we were hosting at her company. I remember her arriving, because she was late and apologetic, saying she was just so busy with work and had lost track of time. When we checked her blood pressure, it was 180/120, far too high. She also told us she had been having headaches and vision problems. When we asked if she had talked to her primary care physician about her symptoms, she said she didn't have one because she was too busy to take the time to find one. We realized we needed to get her treatment right away, though it took a lot of convincing on our part to get her into the ambulance. She had a heart attack while she was in it. It took several weeks for her to get better and get back to work, but thankfully, she did pull through. She had almost died because she hadn't asked for help, hadn't been sure where to turn. And it's not an uncommon story.

We often become so tied up with the day-to-day requirements of our busy lives that we fail to prioritize our most basic need: our own health. Health-care costs are also another big barrier that prohibits many women from utilizing the health-care system. It is estimated that one in four women delayed or went without care due to costs.[9] Considering the limits women have with time and finances, it is important to build a team of professionals you can always and easily turn to and who will help you make the best decisions for your health and well-being.

FACTS YOU NEED TO KNOW

1. The CDC reports that having a regular primary care physician has been associated with lower mortality from all causes, yet nearly 17 percent of women in the US report having no primary care physician.[10]

2. Through routine checkups, primary care doctors can head potentially serious problems off at the pass. As a result, adults in the US who have a primary care provider have 19 percent lower odds of premature death than those who only see specialists for their care.[11]

3. People who have a primary care provider save 33 percent on health care over peers who only see specialists.[12]

4. Many Americans spend less time choosing a physician than they do researching a car before buying one, with 42 percent spending ten or more hours on their next car purchase and 32 percent spending less than one hour researching a physician.[13]

5. According to the US Department of Labor, women make 80 percent of health-care decisions in the United States. Because women are the main medical decision makers, primary care teams know conversations with women can have a significant impact on the health of the entire family.[14]

For all these reasons, you need to take the time to assemble your perfect team!

⚙✳ ESSENTIAL INFO

On your well-being journey, it is important to have a trusted health-care team filled with people who can answer your questions and support you as you make the changes that will lead you to a healthier life. Creating your all-star team requires some groundwork, but the payoff over time will be well worth your effort.

Laying the Groundwork—Finances

If you have health insurance, it is important to understand the plan that you selected. Make sure you understand what's financially covered by your insurance and what isn't. It's not the most exciting reading assignment, but you will be responsible for the "what isn't" and should plan in order to avoid surprising fees. Contact your health insurance provider directly or, if you have insurance through your employer, contact the benefits department to ask for guidance.

Additionally, here are some questions you should know about your health insurance coverage:

1. Which doctors are covered by your plan?
2. Does your plan have a well-being, wellness, or preventive component?
3. Is there a telemedicine option? If yes, what are the fees?
4. Does your plan cover annual eye exams?
5. How frequently can you get a dental exam?
6. Does your plan cover annual skin checks?
7. What prescription coverage do you have?
8. Does your insurance policy have a mental health component? If yes, what does it cover?
9. Do you have a health savings account or health reimbursement account program within your company? If so, do you know how to access it?
10. Are contraceptives covered? If so, which kinds?
11. What should you do if you need emergency care? Is this covered?
12. What if you are traveling out of state and are in need of urgent care?

As you begin to set up your health team, make sure to view your health insurance company's website to review the list of in-network providers. Selecting providers in your network can save you money. If you are trying to select a provider and are having difficulty deciding, most insurance companies provide telephonic support to answer your questions. Give them a call!

If you don't have health insurance, you will either pay for services out of your own pocket or you can tap into some other resources that are available free or at a low cost. See "Appendix 6—Low- or No-Cost Health Resources."

Remember when researching potential health-care providers to focus on those with many reviews. Look for consistently high ratings and pay close attention to posted comments about topics like wait times, willingness to answer questions, and so forth. Below is a list of suggested websites that can help you figure out how various providers rate:

1. Yelp
2. Healthgrades.com
3. Zocdoc
4. AMA DoctorFinder
5. Castle Connolly
6. National Committee for Quality Assurance
7. Physician Compare
8. RateMDs.com
9. Vitals.com
10. U.S. News & World Report

Next I want to share my suggestions for your health team. It may seem like a long list but keep in mind that you certainly do not need them all. Having an understanding of each of these specialists will help you be more informed and reach out for the appropriate care when necessary. This list is separated into two sections: "Must-Have" Resources and "Nice-to-Have" Resources; depending on your insurance and financial resources, you can create the team that works best for you.

"Must-Have" Resources

1. Primary care physician: a physician in internal medicine or family medicine who provides definitive care to the patient at the point of first contact and provides the patient with ongoing/continuous comprehensive care. Primary care physicians provide primary care services, serve as advocates for your care, recommend specialists as needed, and coordinate your use of the entire health-care system. *This is a must-have!*

2. Gynecologist: a physician who focuses on the health of a woman's reproductive system before and after childbearing years. Gynecologists diagnose and treat any conditions concerning the reproductive organs (for example, uterus, fallopian tubes, ovaries, and vagina). They might also treat problems related to the bowel and urinary system, as these are closely tied to the reproductive organs.

3. Obstetrician: a physician who focuses on the health of a woman primarily during pregnancy, childbirth, and immediately following delivery. Obstetricians guide women through pregnancy and childbirth. They diagnose and treat any complications that arise during pregnancy, and they deliver babies vaginally and though cesarean section. *Note: Most gynecologists are also obstetricians, but if you are considering motherhood, you want to ensure your physician is an OB/GYN.*

4. Dentist: a health-care professional who focuses on/ specializes in oral health. Dentists promote oral health, diagnose oral diseases, interpret x-rays, monitor the growth/development of teeth, and perform surgery

on the teeth, tissue, and bones in the mouth. Dentists can also look for signs of oral cancers and spot signs of other health conditions, such as diabetes.

5. Eye specialists: You can select one type of specialist based on your needs.

   a. Optometrist: a health-care professional who provides primary vision care. Optometrists perform vision tests and eye exams. They examine eyes for both vision and health problems, correcting refractive errors by prescribing eyeglasses and contact lenses.

   b. Ophthalmologist: a physician who focuses on medical and surgical care of eyes. Ophthalmologists are the only physicians who can manage the eye/vision care in its entirety. They can prescribe glasses and contact lenses, diagnose and treat eye conditions/diseases, and perform surgery.

6. Dermatologist: a physician who focuses on diseases of the skin, mucous membranes, and hair/nails. Dermatologists diagnose and treat skin conditions including skin cancers, melanomas, and moles. They also deal with cosmetic disorders such as hair loss, effects of aging, and scars.

"Nice-to-Have" Resources

1. Pharmacist: a health-care professional who dispenses prescription medication. Pharmacists help patients achieve optimal medication treatment outcomes while also ensuring that therapy is safe

and cost-effective. They can also recommend reliable over- the-counter (OTC) solutions for less severe health issues.

2. Mental health support: These health-care professionals provide support for mental health issues related to life. Because mental health care needs are broad and unique to each person, the support staff required can vary greatly. It can be a psychologist, psychiatrist, social worker, member of your clergy, or so forth. These different mental health support providers can help with whatever specific issues you are dealing with by providing a safe space for you to talk, teaching you coping mechanisms, informing you of your options, and guiding you through challenging situations.

3. Chiropractor: a health-care professional who treats health problems of the neuromusculoskeletal system (for example, nerves, bones, muscles, and ligaments). Chiropractors use adjustment and manipulation of the spine as well as other clinical interventions to help manage health problems related to the neuromusculoskeletal systems, commonly including neck and/ or back pain.

4. Registered dietitian: a food and nutrition expert who has a college degree and has passed a licensing examination. Registered dietitians help patients/clients improve their health by assessing nutritional needs, offering counseling on nutritional issues, and developing customized nutrition plans. If you have an existing chronic condition (diabetes, hypertension, or so forth), dietitians can be essential in assisting your dietary modifications.

5. Fitness specialist: a fitness professional who focuses on the development and implementation of fitness/exercise programs for clients. Certified personal trainers help their clients improve their health by enhancing their level of fitness and modifying risk factors. To help avoid injury and other issues, make sure to thoroughly research the credentials of your trainer.

6. Phlebotomist: laboratory personnel who draw blood for tests, research, transfusions, or donations. Phlebotomists draw blood from patients/donors but also speak with patients/donors to help them feel less nervous. To avoid causing infection, they help keep work areas and necessary medical instruments clean and sanitary. I recommend identifying where you want to get your labs drawn and utilizing the same facility over time, which will reduce your stress level and save you time researching.

CREATING YOUR HEALTH TEAM WORKSHEET

Use this worksheet as you do your research and start filling in your team. Add their names, addresses, and telephone numbers to have the basics started.

Profession	Name	Research Comments	Contact Information
Primary Care Physician (PCP)			
Gynecologist			
Obstetrician			
Dentist			
Optometrist			
Ophthalmologist			
Dermatologist			

Profession	Name	Research Comments	Contact Information
Pharmacist			
Mental Health Support			
Chiropractor			
Registered Dietitian			
Fitness Specialist/ Certified Personal Trainer (CPT)			
Laboratory Personnel / Phlebotomist			

Once you have your health team in place, take the time to make the most of your appointment by being prepared. Here are some suggestions:

1. Bring a list of all medications (prescription, over-the-counter items, vitamins/supplements, and so forth) with you to your appointment and inform your provider.

2. Keep your personal health and family history handy so that it makes filling out the forms easier and more accurate.

3. Keep track of your menstrual cycle each month and be ready to share the first day of your last period.

4. Have questions prepared in writing before your visit to make the most of the time you have during your visit. There are no silly questions—if you are thinking about something, *ask*.

The bottom line: *You are the only one who can drive your health journey forward. You must confidently speak up, ask questions, and seek the correct medical experts as you need them.*

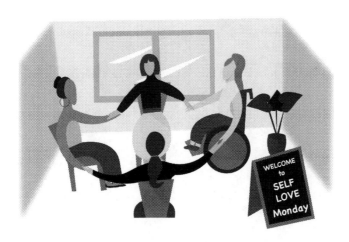

☑️ TAKE CHARGE OF YOUR HEALTH

1. If you still do *not* have a primary care physician (PCP), identify and select one and then make your first appointment.

2. Use your Health Team Worksheet to catalog who is on your current health team and fill in any gaps. Make sure it includes all the professionals in the "must-have" resource section, and if you are missing some, fill in the gaps we listed in this chapter. Be realistic and give yourself the next month to complete this assignment.

3. Research how your current health providers rate. Ask yourself if, with their current rating, you still want them on your team.

4. Make the time to call and get your health appointments lined up for this year. Minimally, contact your primary care physician, gynecologist, and dentist.

BEING YOUR OWN HEALTH WARRIOR

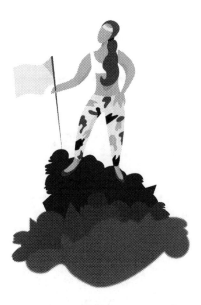

In my opinion, a health warrior is somebody who leads their health care by taking charge and thinking strategically about the best way to get and stay healthy. For this section, I want to tell you the story of a friend of mine because at the time, it genuinely scared us both, so I hope that her story can help inspire you to take the best possible care of yourself that you can. My friend called me a couple of years ago because she wanted my opinion on some symptoms. She had had three urinary tract infections (UTIs) over the preceding twelve months and was also having vaginal itching, increased thirst, and frequent urination. She told me that she only saw her gynecologist and did not have a primary care physician. Her annual gynecological appointments only included pap smears and breast exams but never any blood work. Since she did not have a primary care provider, I told her that she needed to contact the gynecologist, explain her symptoms, and request blood tests immediately.

She listened and took action, and when the results came back, they showed that her fasting blood glucose was 145 (the normal fasting range is less than 100). Her sugar levels were running high, and she had no idea! The in-depth discussion with her gynecologist was helpful too. Apparently, she was also on a birth control pill that contained a type of estrogen that affected her body and how it handled insulin by increasing her blood sugar too.[15] Thankfully, with this new information, she was able to switch birth control methods, change her diet and manage her health in a far more effective way. Six months later, her fasting blood sugar was normal, but more importantly, my friend felt great! This story truly illustrates the importance of knowing your numbers and engaging with your physicians to modify your numbers when necessary—be your own health warrior.

FACTS YOU NEED TO KNOW

1. Chronic diseases are 70 percent related to our lifestyle choices.[16]

2. Heart disease is the number one killer of females, accounting for around 27 percent of all female deaths—killing more women in the US than all forms of cancer combined.[17]

3. The American Heart Association reports that keeping your body mass index (BMI), blood pressure, cholesterol, and blood sugar (glucose) in an acceptable range can improve heart health, reduce the risk of cardiovascular disease, and positively impact your health overall.[18]

4. Although women live, on average, seven years longer than men, they live more years functionally disabled

from stroke, depression, hip fractures, osteoarthritis, and heart disease.[19]

5. John Hopkins Medical Center states, "Forty percent of diagnosed breast cancers are detected by women who feel a lump, so establishing a regular breast self-exam is important."[20]

That is why taking the time and staying in charge of your own health is important!

⚙ ESSENTIAL INFO

Essential actions for achieving and maintaining your health numbers within the desired ranges include regular visits with your health-care providers and routine screenings as necessary based on age. Then you will be able to review the list of recommended screenings and exams broken out by age groups. It may seem like a lot, but now that you have put together your health-care team, lean on them to help you keep all these prioritized! Within each category, you will have the opportunity to come up with your own personal health plan. Over the years in working with clients and for me personally, I have found planning to be a key ingredient for successfully accomplishing these types of health goals.

Now let's think about the different types of screenings you need to get. Here is some helpful information to support you as you plan your annual well-care schedule:

1. **General Health**—Establish your home base by having a primary care physician (PCP). Your PCP can guide your health journey by ordering age-appropriate blood work and monitoring your overall health. It is also helpful to have an established relationship with

this type of health professional for when illness occurs; in most physician practices, current patients will most likely be seen sooner than new patients.

Do you have a primary care doctor? If not, what is your plan for finding one? If you have a PCP, have you scheduled your annual checkup? If you got sick today, who would you call? Take the time now to make your plan to get a PCP and/or schedule your next primary care physician appointment below:

_____

_____

_____

_____

2. **Breast Health**—The American Cancer Society (ACS) has specific recommendations for breast health screening for women with "average risk." Average risk is further defined by not having a personal history of breast cancer, a strong family history of breast cancer, a genetic mutation known to increase the risk of breast cancer (such as in a BRCA gene), and has not had chest radiation therapy before the age of thirty.[21] Here are the specifics:

    Mammogram: This is a low-dose x-ray of the chest. Mammograms can help find cancer early, making it easier to treat.

    - Women ages forty to forty-four have the option to start mammograms every year.

- Women ages forty-five to fifty-four should get mammograms every year.

- Women ages fifty-five and older can switch to mammograms every other year or they can continue annually.[22]

Clinical Breast Exams: This involves having a health professional examine your breasts. According to the ACS, the evidence doesn't support a clear benefit of regular physical examinations to detect breast cancer early when the women are also getting screening mammograms. However, based on age and risk levels, they also recommended considering getting them anyway.[23]

Confused? It becomes complicated in our busy lives to try to figure out at what age to ask our doctors to examine or not examine. My suggestion is that if you are getting your annual checkup, ask your practitioner *every time* to check. It takes less than five minutes! You made the time for the visit; you are already there, and this action can be an extra way to safeguard your health. *Just do it!*

Breast Self-Exams: This involves checking your breasts by feeling and looking on a regular basis. Over the years, the recommendations have changed regarding the importance of breast self-exams, making it difficult for us to figure out what we should actually be doing. Surprisingly, the American Cancer Society also does not recommend regular breast self-exams as part of a routine breast-screening schedule but does recommend it in some situations, as with women in the high-risk categories.[24] Why not err on the cautious side? It *is* your body, and you need to know it and check it—it could be lifesaving for you.

Confused Again? Here is my suggestion. Make an appointment with yourself and check your breasts monthly. If you are still having periods, try to do this three to five days after your period in case you have tender breasts during this time. You can also ask your partner to assist with breast exam support, which can turn into a fun activity too.

There are some great online resources to learn more about how to perform a self-breast exam. Just search "how to perform a self-breast exam" or ask your gynecologist to teach you the basics during your next visit.

Do you have ever-sensitive breasts? Have you felt any lumps? Do you know how to do a self-breast exam? Take the time to make your personal health plan for your breast health below:

_____

_____

_____

_____

3. **Gynecological Checkups**—It is helpful to have regular appointments with your gynecologist and establish consistent screenings as you need them during your lifetime. Here are some guidelines:

   Beginning at age twenty-one, or if you are sexually active, make sure to see your gynecologist annually.

I feel this is a great way to stay on top of your health and any concerns you may be having about your sexual health. If you are thinking about having children or are already a mom, you may want to select an obstetrician/gynecologist.[25]

Based on your age, there are screenings you will need to discuss with your practitioner:

1. Pap test, which screens for cervical cancer. You need to ensure that you get this done every three years. If you have both a Pap smear and human papilloma virus (HPV) test, you may be tested every five years.[26]

2. HPV test, which screens for HPV. HPV is the virus that causes genital warts and several cancers, including cervical cancer.[27]

3. Annual screenings for HIV and other sexually transmitted diseases if you are sexually active.

4. Breast exams.[28]

5. Mammograms.[29]

6. Appropriate blood work that is based on your age and your physician's guidance. Blood work you should request includes a blood sugar test, lipid panel, thyroid-stimulating hormone (TSH) and T4 test, as well as vitamin D levels. You will learn more about these in the screening reference table a little later in this section.[30]

Do you know if your periods are considered normal? If you are sexually active, have you been screened for sexually transmitted disease? Is it painful when you have sex? Is your birth control method safe and right for you? What is your plan for your gynecological health? Take the time to make your personal health plan for this important aspect of your health.

....

....

....

....

4. **Colon Cancer Screening** provides a way to detect colon cancer. Screenings can be performed by using fecal occult blood testing, sigmoidoscopy, or colonoscopy.

   Screening for colorectal cancer begins at age fifty and continues until the age of seventy-five.[31] However, the American Cancer Society recommends that people at higher risk of colorectal cancer start regular screenings at age forty-five. Higher risk means they have a personal history of colorectal cancer or polyps, a family history of colorectal cancer, a personal history of inflammatory bowel disease, or a personal history of getting radiation to the abdomen or pelvic area to treat a prior cancer.[32] *This is another great reason to make sure you get a family health history from your parents if possible; make sure to ask them while you still can.*

Confused Again? My best suggestion is to speak with your primary care physician about this at your annual checkups, listen to your trusted resource, and act accordingly.

Have you thought about your colorectal plan? This one seems odd, but thinking ahead in your life can make a big difference. Have you ever discussed your bowel movements with your doctor? Do you know if your bowel movements are considered normal? Take the time to make your plans for colon cancer screenings or at least a discussion with your physician below:

_____

_____

_____

_____

5. **Skin Checks** provide the opportunity to detect skin cancers or abnormalities.

Experts seem to disagree on how often a person should get exams (annually or when you see a problem area). In my opinion, it is important to examine your skin regularly for changes. If you have a partner, you can ask for some help with this too. If you notice something different—skin or mole changes—contact your dermatologist. I believe as a rule of thumb and to detect problems early, it is important to get annual skin checks. Your primary care doctor can also perform these screenings—all you have to do is ask!

What's your skin care plan to screen for cancer? Do you have any moles or blemishes that concern you? Take the time to write your plan (are you going to see your primary care physician or go to a dermatologist for skin screenings?) below:

----

6. **Dental Checkups** are important to keep your teeth and gums healthy.

   Here is another area where the experts disagree, and it is difficult to get one answer for this question. Keeping your teeth and gums healthy with regular dental visits is important. You should visit your dentist at least once a year. Ideally, if you can, try to go for two checkups each year.

   If you have dental health coverage, take the time to see what is covered in your plan and follow your provider's screening guidelines. If you don't have dental insurance, make sure to get pricing from your dentist on cleanings, x-rays, and procedures. Some dentists will discount the fees if they know you are paying out of pocket, as they will not have to wait for insurance to process the claim.

   What's your plan for your dental needs? Do you have a dentist? Have you seen the dentist in the last year?

Who would you call if you had a toothache? When was the last time you had your teeth cleaned? Write it down and make it happen.

_____

_____

_____

_____

7. **Eye Exams** check your eyes for visual acuity (sharpness), depth perception, eye alignment, and eye movement. Eye exams can provide the first indications of other diseases like hypertension or diabetes. If you have diabetes, hypertension, or a family history of eye disease, it is important to coordinate your eye care with your primary care physician's recommendations.

   If your eyes are healthy and vision is good, you should consider having a complete exam by your eye doctor once in your twenties and twice in your thirties. But at age forty, the American Academy of Ophthalmology recommends that everyone should get a complete eye exam. After your exam, your eye doctor can suggest the frequency of future eye examinations for you based on your needs.[33]

   If you experience an infection, injury, eye pain, or unusual flashes/patterns of light, contact your ophthalmologist for treatment.

   What is your eye care plan? Have you had your eyes checked recently? What would you do if you injured your eye? Who would you call? Take the time to make your health plan for your eye care below:

~~~~~~

~~~~~~

~~~~~~

~~~~~~

8. **Immunizations**—These vaccines protect us from different diseases. As adults, we need a variety of vaccines throughout our lives.

   The flu, a contagious respiratory illness caused by influenza viruses, infects the nose, throat, and sometimes the lungs. It causes mild to severe illness and sometimes can lead to death. The best way to prevent the flu is to get the flu vaccine each year and wash your hands frequently. The CDC recommends a seasonal influenza (flu) vaccine as well as tetanus and/or whooping cough (pertussis) vaccines.[34]

   Have you gotten your diphtheria, tetanus, and whooping cough vaccines? It is recommended that all adults who have never received one get a shot of Tdap. This can be given at any time, regardless of when you last got the tetanus vaccine. This should be followed by either a Td or Tdap shot every ten years.[35]

   The best way to keep track of this is making sure your primary care physician has your up-to-date medical historical records on file. You may also want to have a file of your own—electronic and kept on your phone or kept in a print-based folder at home. Either way, it is your responsibility to keep track too.

It is important to speak with your primary care physician and discuss vaccines based on your age, health conditions, job, lifestyle, and travel habits. The CDC has some great resources to learn more about vaccines. Here is the link to make it easy for you to learn more: https://www.cdc.gov/vaccines/adults/index.html.

Do you know what vaccines you have had? Have you discussed your vaccinations with your PCP? Are you up-to-date with your vaccines? Have you had a flu vaccine? Where would you get a flu vaccine? Take the time to make your personal health plan for your vaccines below:

_____

_____

_____

_____

9. **Osteoporosis Screening**—Osteoporosis is a disease in which the density and quality of bone are reduced. Osteoporosis causes bones to become weak and brittle and most commonly causes fractures in the hip, wrist, or spine. Although this disease affects both men and women of all races, white and Asian women are at the highest risk.[36] Osteoporosis is more common in women, affecting 25 percent of women aged sixty-five and over.[37] Keep in mind that you can prevent or slow the progression of osteoporosis with medications, a healthy diet, and performing weight-bearing exercises that can help prevent bone loss or strengthen already weak bones.[38]

The CDC recommends screening for osteoporosis for women who are sixty-five years old or older or for women who are fifty to sixty-four and have certain risk factors, which include having a parent who has broken a hip. The screening is done performing a bone density test. The results will show whether you have osteopenia or osteoporosis and how suscepti-ble your bones are to fracture.[39]

Now you have a better understanding of the essential num-bers you can use as benchmarks on your journey to better health. Through my career, I have witnessed how knowing health numbers can impact the lifestyle choices we make each day, which ultimately improved our quality of life. Please take your time to understand these different aspects of your health, what they mean to you, the recommended healthy ranges, and what your current numbers are (in the "Your Current Values" column). This information will be valu-able to you as you take future steps toward better health.

Please use this health screening tracker reference table to help you know your values and what they mean.*

Key Metric	What Does It Mean?	Healthy Range(s) for Women	Your Current Values
Body mass index (BMI)	This numerical value takes into account your weight in relation to your height. Value ranges are associated with the following categories: underweight, normal weight, overweight, and obese.	18.6–24.9 indicates a normal weight[40]	
Blood pressure	This refers to the force of blood against your arteries when the heart beats and when it is at rest.	Systolic (top number) less than 120 and diastolic (bottom number) less than 80[41]	
Blood cholesterol	This waxy substance produced by your liver circulates in the blood. Low-density lipoprotein (LDL) cholesterol is known as "bad" cholesterol, as it can build up to cause artery blockage. High-density lipoprotein (HDL) cholesterol is known as "good" cholesterol, as it carries the LDL back to the liver, where it is then removed from the body. Total cholesterol includes both LDL and HDL cholesterol.	LDL cholesterol: less than 70 mg/mL HDL cholesterol: more than 50 mg/DL Total cholesterol: less than 200 mg/dL[42]	

Key Metric	What Does It Mean?	Healthy Range(s) for Women	Your Current Values
Blood sugar (glucose)	This refers to the amount of sugar (glucose) in your blood. Additionally, hemoglobin A1C reflects average blood glucose over the past two to three months.	Fasting blood glucose: less than 100 mg/dL and less than 140 mg/dL two hours after eating Hemoglobin A1C: less than 5.7 percent[43]	

These numbers may vary slightly since most health systems or blood labs have their specific guidelines for the normal values of the numbers listed above. Please speak to your personal care provider to understand what he or she feels is normal for you.

While these exams take time—something in short supply for most of us—getting regular screenings takes less time than treating a disease or condition that could arise if you fail to take preventive action. That means that staying on top of your screenings can ultimately save you a lot of time, not to mention pain and suffering!

☑ TAKE CHARGE OF YOUR HEALTH

1. If you do not have a primary care physician, research and select one; then make an appointment for your annual checkup.

2. Understand your health numbers that you receive from physicians and know if they are in an acceptable range. If not, consider making some lifestyle changes.

3. Get all your necessary screenings scheduled based on your age range and as recommended by your personal care physician.

By now, you can see the importance of creating your own supportive health team and leading your health efforts by taking on the role of being your health warrior. Before you continue reading, please consider taking some time to answer the personal health questions in this part of the book and review/finish all the assignments in the "Take Charge of Your Health" sections.

These assignments were designed to support the next phase of improving your lifestyle, which begins in chapter 3: "Changing Your Daily Habits." I have purposely targeted the most important lifestyle habits you need to consider: hydration, nutrition, fitness, and sleep. Each topic will contain some help for reviewing your status and easy, effective ways to improve your current habits.

3

Changing Your Daily Habits

*Y*our daily health habits affect every aspect of your well-being. In the next five parts, you will learn about the importance of hydration and thinking about your beverage choices, nutrition basics, the keys to getting fit, and the importance of sleep.

═══ STAYING HYDRATED WITH THE RIGHT BEVERAGES ═══

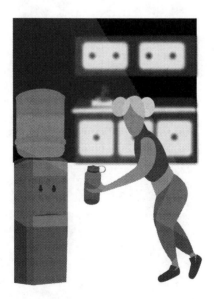

I want to tell you a little secret about myself because this is something my family members and close friends know I am very passionate about. I thought it may be helpful for you to know too—staying hydrated! If you ever meet me, there is a 99 percent chance I will be holding a BPA-free reusable water bottle, which helps me stay healthy by always having water to drink, no matter where or when. I particularly like the transparent ones with numbers on the outside. Seeing how much water is left in the bottle each day at a glance sparks my competitive side and pushes me to finish my daily water requirements. It might seem unusual that I carry this bottle everywhere, but I find it harder to believe that most women don't do this! Many women spend so much time and money hydrating their skin with (often-expensive) products, but we usually don't prioritize hydrating from within, even though drinking water can also help give our skin that beautiful dewy glow. So the next time you reach for a hydration product for your skin in the store, remember to pick up a big BPA-free reusable water bottle too!

FACTS YOU NEED TO KNOW

1. Your brain is 75 percent water, and when you are dehydrated, your brain shrinks which affects your thinking. For women, the general recommended water intake from all food and beverages is seventy-two ounces (nine cups) per day.[44]

2. Dehydrated drivers make twice as many driving errors as hydrated drivers, like the effect of driving while drunk (defined by most states as .08 percent blood alcohol).[45]

3. The average American drinks 450 calories a day. By replacing half of those sugar-loaded beverages with water, you could lose up to twenty-three pounds in a year.[46]

4. According to Statista, Americans drink two cups of coffee per day on average.[47]

5. Approximately 12 percent of adult women report binge drinking three times per month, averaging five drinks per binge.[48]

⚙ ESSENTIAL INFO

An average woman's body is 55 percent water, which includes important body parts such as the brain, heart, lungs, skin, muscles, and kidneys. Your body uses water to maintain its temperature, produce saliva for digestion, lubricate your joints, flush waste from your system, and cushion your brain, among many other things, so it is essential to stay hydrated.[49] Fatigue, headaches, light-headedness, confusion, inability to focus, loss of appetite, increased thirst, dizziness, and muscle cramping can all be signs of dehydration.[50] If you are feeling thirsty, it means your body is already slightly dehydrated. While you may think you consume enough liquids in each day because you drink coffee, tea, soda, and juice, the reality is that there is no substitute for water.

It's true that age, hormone levels, gender, climate, exercise, body structure, and medication all influence our need for water, but there are some general guidelines we should all follow to ensure we stay properly hydrated.

1. Let's start by understanding how much water you need daily. There are two factors to consider when thinking about how much water you should drink daily: your weight and activity levels. As a good rule of thumb, you should try to drink about half an ounce to an ounce of your body weight in ounces of water each day. For example, if you weigh 140 pounds,

you should try to take in at least 70 ounces up to 140 ounces of water (from all of your different noncaffeinated, nonalcoholic beverages) per day.[51] If you know that you will be more active by exercising, you will lose water through your breath as well as sweat and need to follow the guidelines below to replenish the water lost to avoid dehydration.

2. My next helpful tip is to try to start the day with water always. An easy way to ensure that happens is to make a habit of keeping an eight- to twelve-ounce glass of water next to your bed, which you start drinking when you wake up; water by your bed can also quench your thirst if you wake up at night with dry mouth!

3. Additionally, sipping water throughout the day is a good way to prevent dehydration. Your body uses water more effectively when it gets small amounts throughout the day as opposed to your chugging a big glass in the morning and another at night. You should buy a large (twenty-four- to thirty-two-ounce) BPA-free reusable water bottle and carry it with you anywhere, as you do with your phone, so that you remember to drink it. Make it your goal to empty it before lunch and then refill it and drink that before bedtime. You can also make water a part of your meals by drinking eight ounces (one cup) with each meal; this will also help you not overeat and can aid the digestive process.[52]

4. You should also make sure you drink plenty of water before, during, and after any intense activity to replace what was lost through sweat. I try to drink about fifteen ounces of water one to two hours before I begin an intense workout or other activity.

During my workouts, I also drink about eight ounces of water every fifteen to thirty minutes to stay hydrated. Many people turn to a sports drink after a workout, but the reality is that for most of us, water will do the trick to get us back in balance after a workout. Sports drinks have a great deal of sugar and carbohydrates[53] that most of us don't need following our workouts. However, you need to be the judge of electrolyte loss during strenuous activity and decide if you need something other than water.[54]

5. Finally, you may want to ramp up your water intake right before, during, and after your menstrual cycle. The hormones estrogen and progesterone spike at certain times during your monthly cycle and cause you to lose plasma volume. Progesterone can also raise your body temperature, causing you to perspire, and drinking water is one good way to replace any lost moisture.

Regularly drinking water can also lessen the chance of urinary tract infections, as water flushes toxins out of our bodies. It also helps hydrate our skin and improves our bowel functions.[55] Water is a *win-win*!

Remember also that water does not have to be boring. You can change the flavor of your water by squeezing in fresh lemon, lime, or oranges. Cucumber, mint, and frozen berries are also great additions. Sometimes I will pop in a decaffeinated tea bag to add flavor. Be creative! Mix and match fruit and other ingredients for double the flavor.

If you crave more texture, try sparkling water. Just as with tap water, you can jazz up sparkling water with fresh lemon, lime, raspberries, mint, and so forth. If you choose a flavored water, be sure to read the label to identify any added sweeteners and dyes. Be wary of diet sodas, as they contain artificial sweeteners that have been linked to a rise in obesity and diabetes. Brewed herbal teas (without caffeine) are another good option and can be enjoyed hot or cold.

Thinking about What Else You Drink

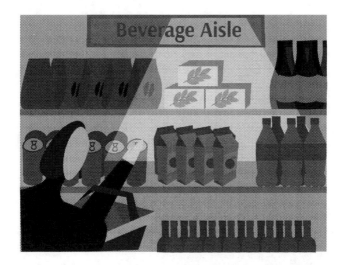

Your beverage choice matters too. A few years ago, I used to start every morning with a big cup of coffee. I would always add three heaping teaspoons of sugar and plenty of sugary flavored creamer. It was like having dessert every morning. A few hours later, my coffee treat would wear off and leave me feeling exhausted. I didn't think much of it at the time, but this fatigue was related to the spike and subsequent fall in my sugar levels and the effects of caffeine. I finally spoke to my physician about it, and he suggested giving up my morning coffee ritual. As far as I was concerned, that was never going to happen! I always looked forward to that treat upon entering the kitchen in the morning. I even used to bring my personal-sized coffee maker on vacations. However, after another year, my blood sugar levels had continued to rise, and with my family history of diabetes, I conceded that I was going to have to change my morning habit.

Believe me, this didn't happen overnight. I first tried modifying my delicious sugar-packed creamer with every other creamer substitute, from almond milk to cashew milk, but it wasn't giving me the same sense of tasteful satisfaction. Therefore, I decided maybe I needed to try a sugar substitute instead to improve flavor. I tried honey, maple syrup, Stevia, and even tried dates to sweeten my coffee, but nothing tasted good to me. Finally, I gave up on coffee completely and decided to try green tea for my morning fix. The first few days were rough when I would enter the kitchen and see my empty coffee space. At first, I felt as if I was missing a dear friend. But as time progressed, I realized it had so many more benefits for me. Green tea also travels easily and is readily available at most restaurants, which has made things much easier for me. Not only does it taste amazing, but it also saves money (no more creamer, coffee, coffee pots needed). The amount of time I now save each morning is priceless because it takes less than two minutes to prepare. Green tea also has many health benefits that include reducing inflammation and preventing cell damage.[56] It took me a couple of weeks to make this adjustment, but honestly, now I am hooked. It was tough to change the habit, but it also left me feeling so much better, so I challenge you to do the same!

Thinking about Caffeine

Caffeine is a stimulant and a diuretic, which will make you urinate more frequently. That means that ultimately, you are going to lose fluid, which will make you less hydrated. While coffee can be a nice way to start your day, be mindful of your caffeine intake. Sources generally agree that taking in up to four hundred milligrams of caffeine per day is safe for most adults, which is equal to about two to four cups of brewed coffee, though during pregnancy it is recommended to keep caffeine intake to less than two hundred milligrams per day.[57] However, due to conflicting recommendations, it is safe to say that less is always better when it comes to caffeine intake. Take time to assess how your body reacts from the caffeine and if you are dependent on caffeine to provide energy; these factors can help guide your decision on how much caffeine you consume daily.

Of course, caffeine is not just found in coffee but also in tea, soda, cocoa, chocolate, and some medications. And given that caffeine content can vary due to the processing and preparation methods of different beverages, I suggest you keep this in mind with respect to your favorite drinks. Here are some common examples to help you get a feel for how much caffeine is in each:[58]

- One eight-ounce cup of coffee: 80 to 100 milligrams
- One twelve-ounce can of cola: 30 to 40 milligrams
- One eight-ounce energy drink: 40 to 250 milligrams
- One eight-ounce cup of green or black tea: 30 to 50 milligrams

It is also important to remember that many prepackaged, commercial, and takeaway caffeinated sports and coffee drinks can additionally contain a lot of sugar and unnecessary calories, so it is always a good idea to look at the nutritional information on those types of beverages before you buy. If you do decide to get a latte, as a rule of thumb, try to keep added sugars to less than ten grams and limit added fat by saying no to things like whipped topping.

What about Alcohol?

Alcohol consumption and abuse is on the rise for women, and it has serious health effects.[59] One study found that the rise in alcohol use in women may be due in part to work-life balance stress.[60] According to the National Institutes of Health, increased anxiety and depression are the leading causes of the increase in alcohol usage.[61] If you do drink, think about your dependence on alcohol and the way it is affecting your life. Do you need to make a change? Why do you drink? If the answer you are thinking is related to mental health stressors (difficult relationships, work stress, depression, and so forth), try skipping forward to the mental health chapter in this book.

If you have a family history of alcoholism and/or currently do not drink, it is not advised to start. Too much alcohol in a diet is associated with weight gain and certain cancers, and it can damage the brain, liver, kidneys, and heart. Moderation, as with everything in our diets, is the key. The Dietary Guidelines for Americans define moderate drinking as up to one drink per day for women. Knowing the amount you drink matters too. Many people do not measure their drinks, and this can lead to heavier pouring. If you are at a restaurant or bar, ask what the quantity is that you will receive. If you are at home, use a liquid measuring cup to fill your glass correctly.

Simply stated, an alcoholic drink is defined as the following: twelve ounces of beer (5 percent alcohol content), eight ounces of malt liquor (7 percent alcohol content), five ounces of wine (12 percent alcohol content), or 1.5 ounces of eighty-proof (40 percent alcohol content) distilled spirits or liquor (for example, gin, rum, vodka, whiskey).[62]

Your genes and your gender influence whether you might become addicted to alcohol, how efficiently you metabolize alcohol, and the effect of alcohol on your organs.[63] In small doses, alcohol changes body chemistry in ways that can reduce heart attacks and strokes. In larger doses, however, it damages many organs, including the heart, brain, and liver, and it damages fetuses in pregnant women. In addition, alcohol addiction plays a key role in traffic deaths and violent crime.[64] Because of gender differences in body structure and chemistry, women absorb more alcohol and take longer to break it down and remove it from their bodies (that is, to metabolize it), causing women to having more long-term health-related problems compared to men.[65]

As for the effect of alcohol on different diseases, more than one hundred studies show that a woman who has one drink per day, compared with a woman who does not drink, has a reduced risk of having a heart attack and the most common kind of stroke. Yet many of these same studies also show that even one drink per day increases a woman's risk of breast cancer.[66] **Confused?** You should be confused because we are getting mixed messages on whether you should drink or not, and at the end of a busy day, for most, usually the drink wins.

You must figure out what is best for you. If you are regularly drinking more than one (measured correctly) alcoholic drink per day, think about making a change. Even the small changes can reduce the negative effects that alcohol can have. The National Institute on Alcohol Abuse and Alcoholism (NIAAA) has some helpful and supportive resources available. Visit https://www.niaaa.nih.gov.

Here are some other ideas that may assist you as you cut back your alcohol consumption:

1. Plan ahead—Take time to write down your daily drinking goals and how many days you plan to drink. Share this with your account-a-buddy (accountability buddy) and try to stick to it.

2. Know how much—Find out how many ounces are being poured into your glass; many bars/restaurants provide "larger pour" sizes; be real and accurate and don't talk yourself into thinking that is okay. It is not.

3. Don't keep alcohol at home—If it is not easily available, you will be less likely to be tempted, and it will provide you with more time to think about your choice to drink if you have to make a special trip to purchase alcohol.

4. Pace Yourself—Sip slowly and consider adding water or club soda to your drink as your glass gets less full. This tip keeps the glass from getting refilled with more alcohol.

5. Space your drinks—If you choose to have more than one drink per evening, think about using a drink spacer: nonalcoholic beverages between alcoholic drinks. Water is a great choice to keep you well-hydrated.

6. Make sure you eat—Many women will skip eating to save calories for alcohol. It is important to remember that alcohol brings no nutrients. Ask yourself, "Am I really making the best choice for me?"

7. Change your environment—Try to avoid places and people in which the main activity is drinking. There are so many great things you can do to replace

drinking time: a fitness program, hobby, or time with friends/family (who don't drink).

8. Feel comfortable saying no to another drink—It is important to practice saying these words confidently. Your true friends will not push you.

9. If you cannot cut down, get some help. Speak to a trusted friend, family member, clergy, or health professional for guidance. You can also contact your local Alcoholics Anonymous; start by calling the national office at (212) 870-3400.

The most important thing to remember about whatever you are drinking is to make sure it's a conscious, healthy choice and that you fully understand the potential health side effects.

☑ TAKE CHARGE OF YOUR HEALTH

1. If you don't own one, buy a large (twenty-four- to thirty-two-ounce) BPA-free reusable water bottle.

2. Start carrying a water bottle that holds at least twenty-four ounces with you everywhere you carry your phone. Fill it at the beginning of the day and challenge yourself to empty it by lunch. Refill it and then drink it again by dinner. *If you are not a fan of plain water, keep a few items on hand to enhance your water flavor: cucumbers, lemon, limes, orange, mint, or berries.*

3. Take time to review your sports drinks, coffee drinks, and others for nutrition information, paying careful attention to the amount of sugar and caffeine in

CHANGING YOUR DAILY HABITS

each; if necessary, make some improvements in your choices to decrease your daily sugar and caffeine. You may recall that the recommended daily allowance (RDA) of sugar is less than twenty-five milligrams daily[67] and the RDA of caffeine is less than four hundred milligrams daily.[68]

4. Think critically about the amount of caffeine you consume and decide if it is healthy or if you'd like to make some changes. If it's the latter, put some of the strategies you learned in this chapter in place to help you decrease your consumption.

5. Think critically about the amount of alcohol you consume and decide if it is healthy or if you'd like to make some changes. *Keep in mind that one drink or less per day is acceptable but not necessary.* If needed, write out some strategies you learned to help you decrease your consumption.

FOCUSING ON NUTRITION

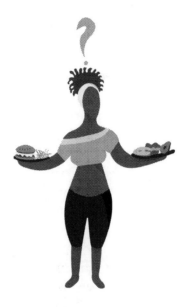

Over the past twenty-five years, I have been involved with the creation and implementation of hundreds of health programs. Two health topics that have been essential components of most of these programs are nutrition and fitness; I have found that almost everyone could do a better job with one or both. Nutrition is a particularly interesting topic because what we put into our bodies makes us look and feel the way that we do. We often focus on food intake for the wrong reasons, such as maniacal weight-loss goals or eating or failing to do so because of emotional strain.

Trying to get my nutrition in the right place has been a life-long journey, and as my life circumstances changed, or the news reports about what's healthy changed, I have tried many different regimes. Ultimately, what I have found is that the most important element of nutrition is thinking about what I eat before I do, for what I put in my body has such a major effect on my health, both mentally and physically.

When I wasn't eating properly, I truly felt the effects. I was feeling aches and pains, was slow to get out of bed in the morning, and was struggling to keep my weight in a range that felt good to me.

However, as I have moved toward healthier food selections, focusing on the foods that make me feel good because they are packed with nutrients, I have noticed that I have more energy, I am sleeping better, and my health numbers, such as fasting glucose and cholesterol count, have improved. This journey has been a major process and didn't happen overnight. It's taken years. This change happened in steps. I first decreased my consumption of processed foods, which included eliminating foods with added fats, sugars, refined starches, and added sodium. The next step, which occurred about a year later, included eliminating dairy and meat from my diet. Then, finally, I was on a plant-based whole food diet. This means that I avoid animal products (like meat, chicken, eggs, and dairy) and focus on plant-based options, which are usually locally sourced and organic. For many, this may seem extreme, but it happens to be what works best for me. I want to make it clear that the takeaway is that balancing your diet in a healthy way that is right for you can make a positive difference in so many aspects of your life! Most importantly, you must find what works best for you in your life.

FACTS YOU NEED TO KNOW

1. Added sugar is in nearly 70 percent of packaged foods, including breads, health foods, snacks, yogurts, and most breakfast foods and sauces.[69]

2. The average American eats about seventeen tea-spoons of added sugar a day—triple the limit for women, which is six teaspoons per day.[70]

3. One in five deaths worldwide is related to consumption of unhealthy foods. Poor diets are also the leading cause of death in the United States.[71]

4. Nearly half of American adults suffer from one or more preventable chronic disease such as cardiovascular disease, high blood pressure, or type 2 diabetes, most due to poor eating patterns and physical inactivity.[72]

5. One in three American adults eat fast food on any given day despite the warnings about its impact on health and obesity.[73]

🔧 ESSENTIAL INFO

The average American puts *one ton* of food in their body each year, so yes, the foods we eat matter.[74] Depending on what you are reading on any given day, there are several different opinions on the types of food we should be consuming, and trying to figure out which suggestions to follow can be confusing and overwhelming. Nevertheless, at the end of the day, what is most important is figuring out what will work best for you and your lifestyle, based on what we know about nutrition from reputable nonpartisan sources.

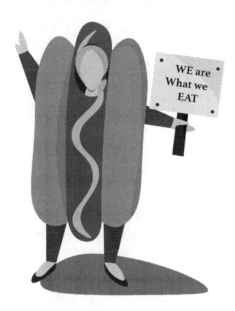

There are so many positive benefits in eating healthfully, and there are some simple rules of thumb we can all follow, like avoiding eating processed foods and foods that contain high levels of sugar and refined flour. Avoid fast and fried foods and try to eat less meat. Instead, focus on plant-based proteins and eat more fruits, vegetables, and whole grains. For more specific rules unique to your needs, you may want to consider working with a nutritionist or registered dietitian. However, before you get that far, you first need to under-stand the science of what you are putting into your body. I know that food science might seem a little boring and clin-ical, but I think it will be helpful for you to better understand the actual chemistry of what we put into our bodies and how it can help you build your case for better food choices.

The Scientific Highlights of Food

Let's cover some important basics. Here are four words that would be helpful for you to understand:

1. Macronutrients
2. Carbohydrates
3. Proteins
4. Fats

1. Macronutrients

Macronutrients are the essential nutrients our bodies need for normal growth and development, specifically carbohydrates, proteins, and fats. In order to gain, maintain, or lose weight, knowing your total caloric needs daily will allow you to gauge the necessary balance of daily macronutrients.[75]

Calculating Your Daily Calorie Needs

The Harris Benedict Equation can help you figure out your individual basal metabolic rate (BMR) and your daily caloric requirements.[76] In order to calculate your specific needs, I suggest going online and searching "Harris Benedict Equation" or "BMI calculator."

Let's say, for example, that you need 1,700 calories per day. Now you need to get the right mix of this equation: CARBS + PROTEIN + FAT = your 1,700 calories.

Women over eighteen years of age should utilize these guidelines and adjust based on their personal weight goals (maintain, lose, or gain):[77]

Carbohydrates	45–65 percent
Protein	10–35 percent
Fat	20–35 percent
Saturated fat	less than 10 percent

The rule I try to follow daily is*:

Carbohydrates	60 percent
Protein	20 percent
Fat	20 percent
Saturated fat	less than 10 percent

*My suggestion is that you experiment with the guideline percentages to come up with what works best by providing the best energy levels for you.

2. Carbohydrates

Carbohydrates are an important source of energy for all cells in our bodies; they are our main fuel source. The carbs we eat plus the amount of insulin we have in our bodies determine our blood sugar levels and have a huge impact on how we feel.

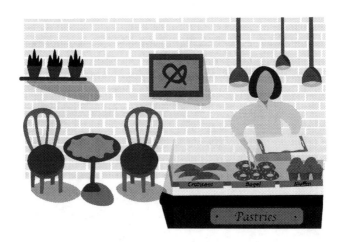

The three carbohydrates we will focus on are starches, sugar, and fiber. Starches—or complex carbohydrates—include starchy vegetables, dried legumes, and grains. Sugars include those naturally occurring (fruit) and added (processed foods). Fiber comes from plant foods.[78]

How should you think about them? When thinking about carbs, make sure you are selecting the right whole grains to get healthy carbs from starchy foods, being wary of sugars and getting enough fiber.

Starch

As for foods that contain starch, here are some examples: starchy vegetables like peas, corn, lima beans, and potatoes; dried beans, lentils, and peas; grains like oats, barley, rice, and wheat. Whole grains are packed with nutrients, including protein, fiber, B vitamins, antioxidants, and trace minerals (iron, zinc, copper, and magnesium). A diet rich in whole grains can also reduce the risk of heart disease, obesity, and some forms of cancer.

Important note: If you choose to buy packaged foods, take the time to read the label! If some of the ingredients are scary (such as dyes and preservatives) and not even possible to pronounce, maybe you should think twice about eating them. Research has shown that some of these ingredients can cause adverse side effects like headaches, palpitations, allergies, and even cancer.[79]

Sugar

Sugars are the simplest type of carbohydrate and are found naturally in fruits and milk, and they show up almost everywhere in most packaged and processed products. The food industry uses sugar to sweeten, prevent spoilage, or improve structure and texture.[80] If you look closely at nutrition labels, you might see sucrose, beet sugar, turbinado, high-fructose corn syrup, dextrose, fruit juice concentrate, corn syrup, cane juice, brown sugar, molasses, and honey, but these are basically just other words for sugar. Thankfully, with the food label design, there is a separate line for added sugars. Since there is no nutritional label on a piece of fruit, you need to remember that they also contain sugar and these sugars need to be factored into your daily allotment.

Your body metabolizes refined sugar and naturally occurring sugars (such as in fruit and milk) differently. Refined sugars are metabolized rapidly, causing insulin and blood sugar levels to skyrocket. Since refined sugar is digested quickly, you don't always feel full after you are done eating (which can lead to eating too much sugar-dense high-caloric foods). The good news about naturally occurring sugars is that along with sugar, they contain fiber, which makes your stomach expand and feel full.[81] Plant foods also have high amounts of fiber, essential minerals, and antioxidants, and dairy foods contain protein and calcium.[82]

An easy way to start improving your diet immediately is by paying attention to added sugars in your own diet. Women should limit their intake of added sugars to no more than twenty-five grams daily (one teaspoon is equal to about four grams). Consuming larger quantities can affect your blood sugar and, when consumed in excess, lead to insulin resistance, cavities, weight gain, and chronic diseases.[83]

Fiber

Fiber aids in digestion, helps with satiety, lowers cholesterol, improves blood sugar levels, and helps people achieve a healthy weight. It also helps reduce the risk for chronic diseases such as obesity, cancers, cardiovascular issues, and diabetes.[84]

Fiber mostly comes from plant foods and is in two forms: soluble and insoluble. Soluble fiber attracts water and will become gel-like during digestion, while insoluble fiber moves things along, assisting with regular bowel movements. Both forms are present in most foods, and our bodies utilize fiber from whole food sources most efficiently.

Fruits and vegetables provide a great dose of fiber. When possible, eat the skin (it has additional fiber benefits too); just remember to clean the skin well before consuming. Fiber is also found in beans and lentils, ground flaxseed, nutritional yeast, whole grains, nuts, and seeds.

Less than 3 percent of Americans get the daily fiber minimums.[85] Women should aim for twenty-five grams of fiber daily.[86] Unfortunately, *our fiber intake is typically too low because of the highly processed and refined typical Western diet*, so if you are like most, you will likely want to increase your intake. It is helpful when buying any type of bread, cracker, or cereal to make sure there is at least one gram of fiber for every ten grams of total carbohydrates by reading the label.

Note that as you increase your fiber intake, it is also recommended to increase your water intake and activity level to help your body adjust to the increased fiber. To help your body adjust, you should only add about five grams of daily fiber at a time and gradually build up to the goal of *at least* twenty-five grams.

What is the typical carbohydrate serving size? Here are some examples of foods that provide about 15 grams of carbohydrates per serving:[87]

> One slice of whole grain bread
> One-half cup of bran cereal

Three cups of popcorn
One-half cup of oatmeal
One-third cup of cooked rice or cooked pasta
One-half cup cooked beans
One small apple, pear, or orange
Two figs

3. Protein

After water, protein is the second most abundant substance in the body. Protein helps grow, maintain, and replace tissue in the body, including muscles, tendons, organs, and skin, as well as enzymes, hormones, neurotransmitters, and other molecules that serve many important functions, and it helps stabilize blood sugar.[88] It is super important!

What else do your need to know? Foods high in protein include soy products, legumes, fish, chicken, meats, and cheese. Remember, protein can be obtained from plant or animal sources. There are benefits to both types, and your choice of protein source should be determined on a personal basis.

Let's start with my personal favorite, plant-based proteins. Plant-based proteins simply means proteins that are free of animal products. There is growing evidence that encourages including more plant-based proteins in your diet for better health; some of these benefits include the following:

- Have anti-inflammation benefits, immunity enhancement, protection from osteoporosis, some cancers, and macular degeneration[89]

- Promote good cardiovascular health and optimize serum cholesterols[90]

◆ Powerfully support digestion through increased fiber intake[91]

◆ Promote weight loss[92]

It will also keep your food costs down because these types of foods are less expensive to purchase in comparison to animal proteins. Finally, there is growing evidence that switching meat products for plants can also help our environment by decreasing the waste from animals produced for food.[93] It's pretty amazing that this one dietary change can positively impact so many factors!

If you get your protein from plant-based sources, ensure you are getting all nine essential amino acids by including a variety such as beans, peas, lentils, nuts, seeds and whole grains.[94] There are also a few plant-based sources that contain all the essential amino acids, like quinoa, soybeans, tempeh, tofu, spirulina, nutritional yeast, rice with beans, pita with hummus, peanut butter sandwiches, chia seeds, and hempseed.[95] With some of these foods, watch your portion sizes to make sure that you stay within your total carbohydrate limit for the day.

If you are interested in learning more about how to make the plant-based conversion, see "Appendix 1—Plant-Based Resources."

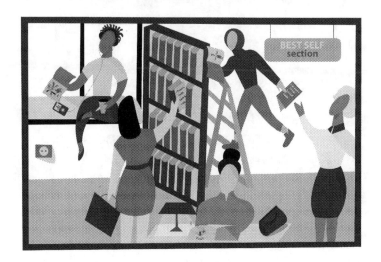

Animal-based proteins are complete proteins with saturated fat and are more commonly eaten in the United States.[96] If you decide to go with this option, try to buy local meat that is grass-fed, free-range, and void of antibiotics. Since animal proteins are higher in saturated fat and contain cholesterol, it's important to think about leaner sources, such as fish, chicken, turkey, egg whites, and game meat such as venison and bison. You can also lower the fat content by purchasing leaner cuts of meat like the loin, sirloin, and chicken breasts. Removing the skin and trimming away visible fat can also help lower the amount of saturated fat you consume. Higher fat and processed meats like bacon, hot dogs, salami, bologna, and sausage contain harmful preservatives and should be eaten no more than occasionally or be eliminated altogether. Research suggests that regularly eating even small amounts of higher fat or processed meats increases your risk of colorectal cancer.[97] So my question to you is whether it's worth the body you love to take a risk. Do you love the taste of bacon more than you love yourself?

Calculating Your Protein Needs and Getting Them

The Dietary Reference Intake is 0.36 grams of protein per pound that you weigh.[98] For example, a person weighing 140 pounds should consume an average of 50 grams of protein per day. But remember you are shooting for 10–35 percent (20 percent is my recommendation) of your total calories for the day.

What about serving sizes? Here are some examples of foods that provide about six to ten grams of protein per serving:[99]

> One-half cup garbanzo beans
> One-half cup tofu
> One ounce of meat, chicken, or fish
> One egg
> Two tablespoons of nut butter
> One-half ounce of mixed nuts

4. Fats

This can be a difficult category for people to understand since not all fats are created equal and they play an important part of maintaining good health. Fat is important to our diet yet has little to no immediate effect on blood sugar; its role is to help with satiety, provide an energy reserve, and allows us to absorb vitamins A, D, E, and K.[100]

How should I think about it? It's simple: healthy fats versus unhealthy fats.

Healthy fats

There are two groups of fats that are known to be heart healthy and may help with lowering LDL cholesterol, improving insulin levels, improving glucose levels, and re-ducing inflammation. These groups are called monounsat-urated fats and polyunsaturated fats.[101] Here's a little more information about each:

1. *Monounsaturated fats* are all plant-based. Sources include olive, canola, peanut, and sesame oils as well as avocados, cashews, peanuts, nut butters, and other cooking oils made from plants.[102]

2. *Polyunsaturated fats* may or may not be plant-based. Sources include chia seeds, flax, walnuts, fatty fish (salmon, tuna, trout, herring, sardines, and mackerel), and tofu. Polyunsaturated fats also include foods with omega-3 and omega-6 fatty acids. Additional omega-6 sources include poultry, nuts, and acai.[103] Polyunsaturated fatty acids are essential for a healthy diet and help reduce the risk of heart disease. Having a variety of these foods in your diet is essential for good health.[104]

Unhealthy fats

There are also two groups of fats that are known as un-healthy: trans fats and saturated fats. To reduce your risk of heart disease, improve HDL cholesterol levels, and decrease your risk of other chronic conditions, it's very important to *limit* your daily consumption of trans fats and saturated fats.[105]

Trans fats are a byproduct of hydrogenation, which is a pro-cess that turns healthy oils into solids to prevent them from spoiling. Trans fats can be found in packaged or boxed foods, coffee creamers, stick margarines, shortening, most fast-food french fries, and baked goods.[106]

Saturated fats are fats that are mostly solid at room temperature. Common sources of saturated fats include red meat, whole fat dairy, butter, ice cream, lard, and tropical oils. The US Dietary Guidelines recommend eating no more than 10 percent of your total daily calories from saturated fats.[107]

Trans fats and saturated fats are sometimes intertwined

Trans fats are listed on food labels under saturated fats and can be listed as a "0" if the product has less than half a gram per serving.[108] If that's the case, check the ingredients for partially hydrogenated oils. If your product contains a partially hydrogenated oil, that means it contains some small amount of trans fat. If this is a food product you use daily (like a coffee creamer), that little bit of extra fat each day adds up to a lot over the course of a year!

Trans fats also occur naturally in some meats and should be limited in your diet. Trans fats can also create inflammation, which is linked to heart disease, stroke, diabetes, and other chronic conditions.[109] Since the FDA has cracked down on the food industry and has required most trans fats to be eliminated from foods, food manufacturers have replaced this ingredient with coconut, palm kernel, and other palm oils. The problem is that these replacements are *still fats* that aren't good for you because they contain saturated fat and are still packed with calories.[110] They may taste good, but your body will pay the price over time.

I suggest that you seriously look at the labels of the foods that you eat. If any of them contain trans fats, eliminate them from your diet. *It's not worth the health risk!* You also need to make a conscious effort to read the ingredients and decide if this is what you want to put into your body. Track your saturated fats, too—remember, you are aiming for less than 10 percent per day of your total calories.

Talking with a registered dietitian and knowing your current biometric numbers are good ways to determine if the quality or quantity of fat in your current diet is appropriate.

A few other nutritional components to keep in mind:

1. **Salt:** It adds flavor to food but also has its downsides: it also contributes to raising blood pressure and impairs your artery function.[111] The 2015–2020 US Dietary Guidelines on sodium intake is 2,300 milligrams or less per day.[112] Be mindful of your consumption of processed and prepared foods, as they typically contain high levels of salt and additives. Also be on the lookout for *lots of extra salt* in restaurants. Everyone knows eating salt makes us thirsty. Many restaurants add additional salt to foods for flavor and to make more money on drinks (adding salt will make you thirstier).[113]

2. **Calcium:** To maintain bone health, the recommended dietary allowance (RDA) for calcium is 1,000 milligrams for women ages nineteen through fifty and 1,200 milligrams for women aged fifty-one and older.[114] The best sources of calcium are often fortified beverages such as cashew, almond, and soy milk. Calcium is also found in dark green leafy vegetables, dried peas and beans, fish with bones, and calcium-fortified juices and cereals.[115] If you choose dairy products for calcium, make sure they are organic to avoid contaminants.[116]

3. **Fruits and Veggies:** Adequate intake of fruits and vegetables has been linked to a lower risk of developing several chronic health conditions, including heart disease and cancer.[117] Increased fruit and vegetable intake can also help replace calorie-dense processed

foods. The recommended daily intake of fruits and vegetables is as follows:[118]

Fruit: 1-1/2 cups—fresh, frozen, canned, or dried, without added sugars

Vegetables: 2-1/2 cups—fresh, frozen, or canned, without added salt

A few tips I use when enjoying fruits and veggies:

- To reduce pesticides and support sustainably produced foods, buy organic when possible. Organic foods are labelled and guaranteed by the US government to have been produced following specific guidelines.

- Try to find seasonal and locally grown produce to avoid buying foods that have been picked unripe and shipped for weeks to get to the store.

- When I unpack my groceries, I wash all fruits and veggies with one teaspoon of mild soap/gallon of water before storing; it's super important to wash all skins before cutting to avoid eating contaminants!

Behavioral Insights to Support You

Are you trying to be healthy, lose or gain weight, feel more energetic, and/or sleep better? Making these small changes in your eating habits will lead to big improvements in your overall health. Set specific nonrestrictive goals and just try to improve things bit by bit or bite by bite.

Keep in mind that no one is perfect. You will set yourself up for failure if you think perfection is the only solution. *Love your current body and be kind to it as you practice making it a healthier version of you.*

Many of us use food as our friend to deal with emotions and unpleasant memories; if this is the case, try working on those underlying issues as part of your transformation plan.

The goal is to move toward healthier food choices in a gradual and manageable way. It took you years to get to where you are today, and change takes time. Commitment, planning, and practice will lead you to success when it comes to making healthy eating a lifetime habit.

In order to change behavior, it is often helpful to identify the reasons behind these changes. Take the time to write down the reasons you want to improve your eating habits:

_____

_____

_____

_____

_____

_____

_____

Now that you have identified the reasons to improve your eating, write down what you are willing to do to begin making changes. Examples could include using a list to plan meals, eliminating (name specifics) from my kitchen, packing lunches to avoid fast food, and so forth.

_____

_____

_____

_____

_____

_____

_____

It's time to enlist your team; who you will have on your support team? Examples could include your partner, close friend, roommate, family member, registered dietitian to provide accurate guidance, psychologist to work on underlying issues or an account-a-buddy to share your feelings.

_____

_____

_____

_____

_____

_____

Get Your Kitchen Ready!

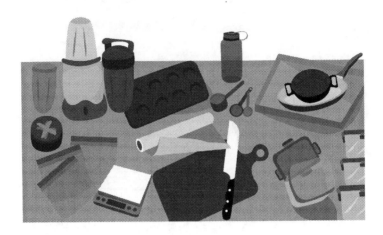

Kitchen aids: Once you have committed to making some dietary improvements, it is important to be prepared with the right kitchen aids to assist you in making meal prep easy and fun. My suggestion is for you to assess your current kitchen and gather the items below. If you do not have all of them, make the investment in yourself:

1. Measuring cups, spoons, and a food scale* to keep you honest with your portions

2. Insulated lunch bag and ice packs to help you be prepared for work and outings

3. Glass to-go containers for storing foods and taking leftovers to go

4. Strainer for rinsing rice, washing berries, or straining noodles

5. Muffin tins, baking sheets, and pie pans to prepare yummy treats

6. High-powered blender to make smoothies, salad dressings, and chop nuts/seeds

7. Food processor—super helpful for creating great recipes that require processing larger amounts

8. Electric mixer—a handheld one will work just fine

9. Toaster—try to get one with different settings (bagel, English muffin, bread) to take the guesswork out of which setting to select

10. Cutting boards, one for produce and another one for meats/fish

11. Slow cooker—easy to prepare meals ahead and great to come home to after work

12. Other items to consider: can opener, citrus zester, grater, pizza cutter, potato masher, tongs of various sizes, veggie peeler, wire whisks and a variety of knives for cutting, parchment paper, and nonstick foil

*Measuring your food: When you measure your food, you will not only learn a lot about portion control, but you can also better manage what you eat. You don't have to measure forever, just until you get the hang of correctly eyeballing your portions. It may seem like a pain and you don't want to take the time, but I know from experience that it helps manage your eating much more effectively. Just do it.

Once you have some achievable goals in mind and your cupboard is ready to go, here are some simple shopping tips you may want to consider:

For meals, remember that grilling, baking, broiling, steaming, slow cooking, and sautéing can be healthy options, especially when you add the right herbs, sodium-free seasonings, and marinades. When using your slow cooker sautéing, remember to limit the fat additives to keep your dish healthier for you. A fresh-squeezed lemon or lime can bring life to a meal. As you make your grocery list, remember to add your spice selections.

Planning meals ahead starts with recipes! To get you started, I have a list of some great places to get some new recipe ideas (see "Appendix 2—Recipe Resources).

Are you up for trying something new to eat? Take the time to list three healthy recipes you plan to make this month below:

....

....

....

....

Think before buying: I have a saying: "If it's not in your house, it won't end up in your tummy." The grocery store is the place to begin making healthier food choices. I also suggest sketching out your meal plan for the week—breakfast, lunch, and dinner. Try to prepare foods the night before to avoid hurrying in the morning and reduce morning stress.

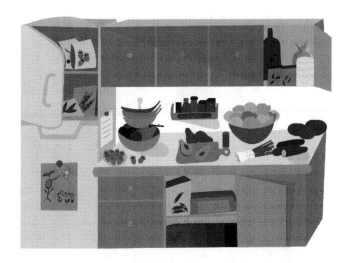

Go into the store with a list and stick to it! Shop the perimeter of the store, where you will find produce and whole grains and not a lot of the less healthy food options. While shopping, keep in mind that there is no such thing as a food you can eat an infinite amount of and still be healthy. The best strategy is to understand what a balanced meal looks like in terms of carbohydrates, protein, and fat—incorporating these into a weekly plan.

Here are some basics you may want to have in your kitchen at all times to help you be prepared:

1. Three to five different fresh fruits of choice—pick at least one type of berry

2. One to two frozen fruits of choice for smoothies

3. Three to five different fresh vegetables of choice

4. One to two frozen vegetables of choice

5. Avocados are a must—I always have two to four in the kitchen

6. Dates are great for a snack or for baking

7. One to two salad bases (such as spinach, arugula, spring mix)

8. A variety of spices (if possible, buy organic):

   Allspice
   Basil
   Bay leaves
   Cayenne
   Chili powder
   Cinnamon
   Cumin
   Dill
   Garlic powder
   Ginger
   Ground nutmeg
   Ground onion powder
   Oregano
   Paprika
   Pepper
   Rosemary
   Saffron
   Sage
   Tarragon
   Thyme
   Vanilla extract

9. Grains: farro, whole wheat pasta, brown rice, quinoa, rolled oats, whole wheat pita, rice cakes, whole grain bread, whole wheat tortillas

10. Nuts/seeds: almonds, hazelnuts, cashews, peanut and almond butter, flaxseed, hempseed, chia seeds

11. Your protein source: tofu, tempeh, beans (kidney or black), lentils, or animal-based of choice

12. Almond, cashew, or some other form of nondairy milk—great for recipes and smoothies

13. Low-sodium vegetable broth

14. Light coconut milk for cooking

15. Hot sauce without added sugar

16. Nutritional yeast—great for flavoring and has protein

Keep in mind to read labels and follow our earlier discussed guidelines. Avoid added sugars and try to buy organic, if possible.

Do you plan your meals? What is in your kitchen to-day? What do you need to improve? Healthy eating starts with the right ingredients. Take the time to write your grocery list below:

_____

_____

_____

_____

_____

Now that you've brought healthy food items home, you need to do something with them or they will just go to waste in your refrigerator. If you didn't wash your produce when you unpacked your grocery bags, spend ten to fifteen minutes at the beginning of the week washing, cutting, and putting veggies into individual servings so that when you need a snack, you can just grab a healthy one. This process works for most vegetables and some fruits so use your discretion. My point is that planning and preparing ahead will save you time and eliminate excuses for not grabbing a healthy option each day. I use my Saturday or Sunday afternoons for this task and often enlist help from the family to get the job done quicker and help make everyone aware about the healthy options available in our fridge. To keep fresh-cut vegetables crispy, try putting a slightly damp paper towel on top of them in the sealed container; this helps absorb moisture.

Keeping Track of Your Success

Don't forget to track your intake—this is essential for success. It may sound difficult at first, but it can become a useful habit for you to ensure that you are getting the right amount of food and nutrients to keep your body at its best. Tracking can be done in your journal or on one of the many applications available today. Apps are very helpful because many are free and they help you see the daily picture, which includes your percent of fat/carbs/protein, macronutrients, vitamins, calories, fiber, and more. App sources are listed in "Appendix 3—App Sources for You."

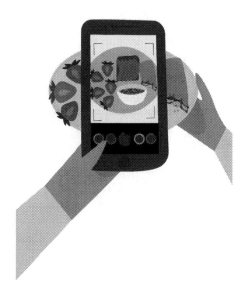

As you move toward healthier nutrition goals, be conscious about portion control. Your food scale, measuring tools, and tracking apps can help, but what about your thoughts? Here are easy planning tips to help you not overindulge:

1. Next time try walking away when you feel satisfied but not stuffed. A good way to do this is to use the "plate and put back" technique. Take your normal portion and then put two tablespoons of it back in the serving dish.

2. Another tip you can try is to switch to smaller plates, like appetizer or salad plates, to help reduce portion size and make it look as if you have more food on your plate.

3. To avoid hunger, include a lean protein source and fiber with each meal, as it will keep you fuller for a longer period.

4. It is also interesting to note that our hunger cues are stronger than our thirst cues, so many times when you think you are hungry, you could just be thirsty. Next time you feel hungry, drink a full glass of water and then wait a little while to see if you really are hungry or if what you thought was a hunger cue turned out to be just a cry for water.

5. Remember not to eat too quickly. Eating fast allows us to take in more calories than we actually need, before our bodies can send us the cue that we are full. Try putting your utensils down between bites.

6. Finally, use all your senses before you begin eating to help you slow down. That means no eating while cooking, watching television, or finishing leftovers off the kids' plates. Take the time to enjoy—appreciating the aroma, look, and taste of the food can enhance your dining pleasure! Look at all the colors on the plate. When you take a bite, what flavors can you taste? Digestion starts in your mouth so chew your food well.

I can almost guarantee that you did not get to your current nutritional habits overnight, and you will not make these suggested changes in one day. Be patient and kind to yourself and celebrate your progress, but keep pushing yourself forward to better health; it takes commitment and practice.

✅ TAKE CHARGE OF YOUR HEALTH

1. Use the resources provided to calculate your daily macronutrient needs and set goals for how much carbohydrate, protein, fats, fiber, sugar, and so forth, you would like to consume.

2. Take the time to download a nutrition app that allows you to track your food. Make notes in the app about which meals make you feel good and which make you feel bad. Look back at your notes and make changes accordingly.

3. Take the time and purchase a food scale and measuring cups and then commit to using these tools until you can correctly eyeball correct portion sizes.

4. Identify your nutritional support team by making your list and ask those people for help. The people in your life who are the most motivating and supportive will be there for you in good times and times that you really need them. Changing your eating habits is not easy, and if you live with someone, changing your eating habits can be positive motivation on days you are struggling to keep up with your goals. Celebrate your successes and learn from your setbacks.

MAINTAINING SUSTAINABLE FITNESS

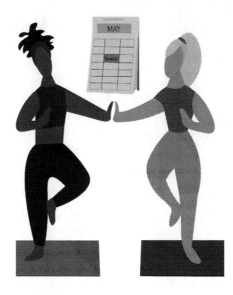

As I mentioned in the "Focusing on Nutrition" part, fitness is another key component for great health. There are so many benefits from being fit, which I will discuss with you shortly. Over the years, I have often been asked what the best exercise is; my standard response is the one that you enjoy doing and will practice regularly! One of the consistent roadblocks for many is finding the time. Personally, I try to plan my upcoming week each Sunday, and that always includes specific blocks of time for fitness. When our sons lived at home, I used to include them in the plans too. I have so many fond memories of us all staying fit together. These days my accountability buddy or, as I call him, my account-a-buddy, is my husband. We make sure fitness is always a part of our day (even if we are traveling) because it is truly the daily prescription for good health. I would encourage you to do the same, planning your time for fitness and sticking to it! Someone once commented to me about how committed I am to my fitness regime and asked what I was training for ... It took me less than three seconds to respond with the word *life.* If you truly commit to doing that, it'll make a world of difference and won't be viewed as a chore but something that you will look forward to doing for you.

 FACTS YOU NEED TO KNOW

1. Regular physical activity can help lower the risk of high blood pressure, heart disease, stroke, type 2 diabetes, and unhealthy cholesterol levels. It can also help with mental and emotional benefits such as decreased stress and improved mood.[119]

2. More than 60 percent of American women do not engage in the recommended amount of physical activity; more than 25 percent are not active at all.[120]

3. Only one in three adults receive the recommended amount of physical activity each week.

4. Physical inactivity is more common among women than men.[121]

5. Social support from family and friends has been consistently and positively related to regular physical activity.[122]

ESSENTIAL INFO

For exercise to be truly effective, you need to make time for it and schedule it as part of your everyday routine for the long term. I have found that if you identify the reasons you want to be fit, it will help you realize that it is worth making time for it. I'd like you to take some time to write down what you want to accomplish by being fit. Are you trying to be more flexible, improve your mood, manage stress, sleep better, improve your health metrics (body mass index, blood pressure, and so on), tone your body, spend fun time with your family, lose weight, or increase your stamina?

What are your reasons for wanting to stay fit or get fit? How would a fitness regime improve your life? Take some time to think and then write out three to five reasons you want to be fit:

_____

_____

_____

_____

It will be super helpful to remember those goals and come back to them often to help remind you why you are prioritizing exercise.

Getting Everyone on Board

It's okay to put yourself first when it comes to fitness and hold your exercise time as sacred. When you do that, you'll find you have more energy to give to others who need things from you or rely on you. If you are having trouble making the time, be creative and enlist your support team. If you can't convince them to exercise with you, ask them to support you in your efforts. It may also help you to find an "account-a-buddy" who can work out with you and help provide motivation! Your support system will help you keep on track with your exercise program.

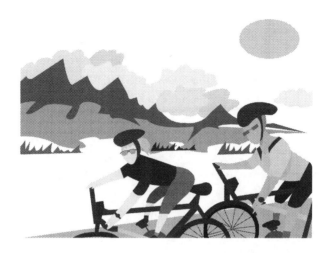

Perhaps the biggest bonus from exercising goes beyond the physical body; improved mood, decreased stress, decreased depression and anxiety, increased energy, and an improved overall quality of life could be the biggest benefits you get from exercising on a regular basis, all of which benefit the people around you as well.[123] So make sure your support team reminds you that you are doing this for all of you! Also, remember that you don't need to stick to just one type of exercise or follow the same exercise routine each time you work out. Get creative. In fact, switching things up can be very beneficial to achieving your exercise goals. In addition, it's a lot more fun!

Do you feel supported by your current circle of family and friends? Who do you want on your support team as your account-a-buddy (ies)? Write their names below:

Some General Guidelines for Staying Fit

You may be wondering how to come up with fitness goals in the first place. Well, let's start by looking at some general guidelines:

1. Women need to do at least 150 to 300 minutes a week of moderate intensity, or 75 minutes to 150 minutes a week of vigorous-intensity aerobic physical activity, or an equivalent combination of moderate and vigorous intensity aerobic activity:[124] Moderate intensity is defined as an increase in heart rate while still being able to comfortably hold a conversation. Examples include brisk walking, water aerobics, biking (slower than ten miles per hour), and playing doubles tennis.[125] Vigorous intensity is defined as significant increase in heart rate, where breathing inhibits the ability to hold a conversation. Examples include power walking, jogging, running, biking (ten miles per hour or faster), playing singles tennis, and uphill hiking.[126]

2. Women should strength train all major muscle groups twice per week with moderate to high intensity. However, more than 80 percent of adults do not meet the guidelines for recommended aerobic and muscle-strengthening activities.[127]

3. Women who are pregnant should stay under the care of their health-care provider, who can monitor the progress of the pregnancy. It is also important to check with the health provider on how to adjust physical activity during pregnancy and after the baby is born.[128]

I know this may all sound complicated and difficult to fit into your life ... I get it. It is a lot to think about with your other responsibilities—family, work, and community. That's why 80 percent of women (as I mentioned in our facts earlier) are not active. Plan to start in small increments each day and work your way up.

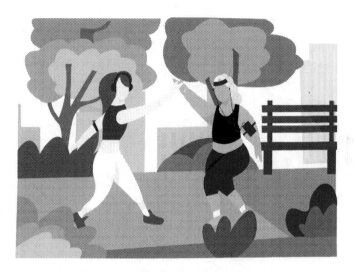

Before you begin any fitness program, it's important that you check with your doctor to ensure you are well enough to start. Chat with him or her about what you are planning to do in order for that person to make an informed decision. Once you get the okay from your doctor, it's time to get started! The good news is that there is no one-size-fits-all exercise program. You'll get the biggest benefit from exercise programs that are customized to meet your needs.

Creating Your Own Personalized Plan for Exercise

Your goal with fitness should be to create a sustainable fitness program. In order to do this, it is very helpful to use the FITT (frequency, intensity, time, and type) Principles to guide your success. Health and fitness professionals have used these concepts for many years.[129]

Frequency: This refers to how often you exercise per week. Start slowly if you are new to exercising and work up to working out more days per week as your body becomes accustomed to an increased level of activity.

Intensity: This is how hard you work out. Again, lower intensity to start, increasing as you progress. Doing too much too soon can lead to injuries, and that is *not* sustainable. When it comes to making exercise a lifelong habit, slow and steady is the way to go. Knowing your target heart rate is important too. I suggest learning how to check your pulse to track your heart rate. It's easy to do and costs nothing.

As for target heart rate, the Karvonen formula is a way to determine your target heart rate. Target heart rate equals maximum heart rate minus resting heart rate times percent of intensity plus resting heart rate.[130] To measure your resting heart rate, use the tips of your first two fingers (not thumb) to press lightly over the blood vessels (pulse) on the thumb side of your wrist. Count your pulse for ten seconds and multiply it by six to find your beats per minute. Your maximum heart rate is 220 minus your age. For example, the maximum heart rate for a twenty-nine-year-old woman is 191 (220 minus 29 equals 191). The American Heart Association recommends the following target heart rate zones depending on your intensity:[131]

- Moderate exercise intensity: 50 percent to about 70 percent of your maximum heart rate
- Vigorous exercise intensity: 70 percent to about 85 percent of your maximum heart rate

There are many instructional online videos that can demonstrate the correct technique for checking your heart rate; search "how to check your pulse" and you get you some great responses. If your budget permits, I highly recommend investing in a heart rate monitor that can measure them for you. It makes it much easier to track your heart rate during your workout time. *Remember that I am all about making your life easier!*

Time: This refers to how long you exercise. You are shooting for 150 to 300 minutes per week of moderate intensity or 75 minutes to 150 minutes per week of vigorous-intensity aerobic physical activity or an equivalent combination of both.[132] However, it is important to start with less time if you have never exercised or are returning to exercise after a prolonged absence. Ease into your time but work to achieve the recommended amounts.

Type: There are a variety of ways to exercise that include cardio, muscle strength, muscle endurance, and flexibility. To get the maximum benefit from your exercise program, include all types over the course of a week. Also, always be sure to listen to your body; it will tell you when to push and when to slow down, stop, or reduce intensity. Never work out if you are experiencing pain that could be an injury.

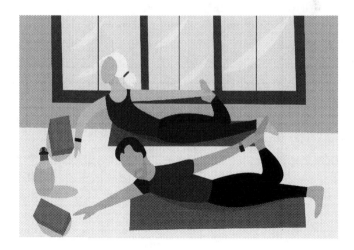

More Health Benefits of Your Fitness Program

When you engage in exercises that fall into the cardio cat-egory, your entire body will benefit; you'll see improvements in your body's overall efficiency. All the systems in your body will thank you for getting on the treadmill, bike, or elliptical—or even taking a vigorous walk.

If you want to improve muscle and bone strength, as well as improve your endurance and stamina, you need to mix resistance training into your exercise routine. Weights and re-sistance bands are great ways to give your muscles a work-out. Being flexible is important, no matter how old we are, but as we age, flexibility becomes critical. Improved range of motion in joints, overall stability, less muscle soreness, and a reduction in the risk of accidents are the main benefits of improved flexibility.

At the beginning of your exercise program, check your measurements and your body fat percentage to provide a measurable metric. Those are better indicators of success than what the scale is telling you. Remember that muscle is denser than fat and may increase the weight on the scale even though you will be trimming down.[133] There are other ways to see if you are benefiting from your fitness program: focusing on how you feel, your energy level, and your moods.

I also suggest that you keep a record of your workouts and look back on them to see your progress. Notice things like frequency improvements, time improvements, and so forth. If you can, use an app to help keep you on track. MyFitnessPal (which tracks your nutrition too) and Apple Watch Health are great resources for tracking.

I have also included a list of some great fitness program apps in "Appendix 4—Fitness App Resources for You."

Check these out and select what works best for you. These on-demand resources allow you to work out on your schedule in your space with your equipment of choice, which helps you stay excuse-free! You can stretch, do cardio, practice yoga, strength train, and more with these fun and innovative programs.

> *As mentioned several times, and probably to the point of getting annoying, planning is key. Take the time to write out three to five ways you plan to improve your current fitness level. You may want to include adding exercise activities on your calendar for better planning.*

_____

_____

_____

_____

Finally, it is important to celebrate your achievements and reach your short- and long-term goals. Rather than using food as a reward, treat yourself to a new book, something for your exercise wardrobe, a healthy picnic in the park, or something else that helps you celebrate your wins. You deserve to take time to feel good and to celebrate yourself for doing so!

✅ TAKE CHARGE OF YOUR HEALTH

1. Think and determine the types of exercise you prefer. Finding what you like will make it easier to stick with exercise.

2. Make a list of the areas of your life and the people in it who will be positively affected by the impacts of exercise on your mood, stress levels, and energy. *Your name* should be first.

3. Identify your support team, the people in your life who are the most motivating and supportive. Work out with them or ask them for help with motivation on days you are struggling to keep up with your goals.

4. Create an exercise plan to improve your current fitness level (can be digital or on paper). Jot down your short- and long-term goals. Log your workouts, including what you did, how long you did it, how you felt, and so forth.

GETTING ENOUGH SLEEP

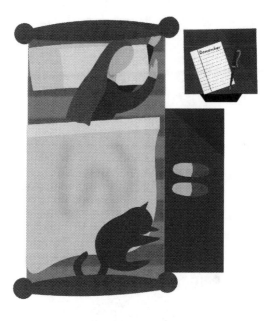

In my working career, the topic of sleep deprivation and the effects on well-being came up constantly. In my conversations with women, it seemed that often they didn't see the genuine benefit of sleep. Sleep was viewed as something that is easy to give up in order to prioritize our to-do lists. Throughout my life, I have made this mistake too, but it is not something to take lightly.

A few years ago, during the busiest time in my career, I was in a meeting and I tried to make a comment, but my speech came out garbled and unintelligible. That day, I had also been struggling with dizziness. In that moment, I genuinely thought I was having a stroke. I reached out to my primary care doctor, and of course they had to run all kinds of tests, thinking that if not a stroke, perhaps I had some other serious problem, perhaps a brain tumor. Thankfully, all the tests came back negative, but I was at a loss for what was wrong with me. Finally, one of the specialists (a neurologist) asked me how much I was sleeping per night. My answer at that time was about four to six hours. She then told me that my sleep patterns were the culprit behind my symptoms and that the only way to ensure my body was properly repairing itself was to get enough sleep each night. I realized then that I could not continue to reduce sleep to make time for other things, as sleep is a necessity. I could finally give myself permission to sleep. It still was not an immediate change; it took me months to fix my sleeping patterns fully, but I am a far healthier woman to this day for it. I learned the hard way that adequate sleep is important to physical health, as sleep is involved in healing the heart and blood vessels, maintaining healthy levels of hormones, and supporting the immune system.

 ## FACTS YOU NEED TO KNOW

1. According to the American Academy of Sleep Medicine, the recommended amount of sleep for adults is at least seven hours per day.[134]

2. Because women tend to expend more mental energy during the day while multitasking, it has been estimated that women require about twenty more minutes of sleep per day than men do.[135]

3. More than one in three Americans do not meet the recommended sleep duration on a regular basis.[136]

4. The National Sleep Foundation reports that women are twice as likely to suffer from insomnia as men are. The changing levels of hormones in the body due to menstruation, pregnancy, and menopause can be associated with inadequate sleep.[137]

5. According to the Centers for Disease Control and Prevention, sleeping fewer than seven hours per day can lead to an increased risk of developing several chronic health conditions such as high blood pressure, depression, type 2 diabetes, hypertension, coronary heart disease, and obesity.[138]

⚙✳ ESSENTIAL INFO

As you can see by now, sleep is an extremely important component of a person's overall health. The American Academy of Sleep Medicine and the Sleep Research Society recommends that adults aged eighteen to sixty years of age sleep at least seven hours each night to promote optimal health and well-being. Sleeping fewer than seven hours is associated with an increased risk of developing chronic conditions such as obesity, diabetes, high blood pressure, heart disease, stroke, and frequent mental distress.[139] Women are more likely to have trouble sleeping at night and excessive daytime sleepiness than men are. Women also have a higher degree of difficulty concentrating and remembering things due to sleepiness or tiredness.[140] Adopting healthy sleep habits is an easy way for you to improve your physical health, brain function, and emotional well-being.[141]

Insomnia manifests in two ways: either you can't fall asleep or you fall asleep but then wake up in the middle of the night, only to discover you can't fall back asleep. If you have had these issues, you have probably wondered why you aren't sleeping properly and then you lose more sleep worrying. Here are some simple things you can start now to make it easier to sleep:

*   **Follow a routine**: If possible, go to bed at the same time every night and wake up at the same time every

morning.[142] It may also help to take a shower right before bed to help yourself relax and train your body that showering comes right before sleeping. Or you could perhaps do something relaxing like reading, listening to music, or meditating to prepare you for sleep. **If you have children, get them on a routine too.**

◆ **Avoid sleeping in**: Unbelievably, consistently waking up within fifteen to twenty minutes the same time each day will help you sleep better at night because it maintains a regular rhythm for your body.[143]

◆ **Prepare your bedroom—make it a sleep sanctuary**: Make sure the bedroom is cool and well ventilated. Remove clutter and make it visually calming. Invest in room-darkening shades; they are well worth it. Sleep on a firm mattress. Mask disruptive noise with a fan, white noise, or soothing nature sounds. In addition, I use a lavender scent on my pillow to help fall asleep each night, which works incredibly well.

◆ **Avoid light at night**: If you wake up to go to the bathroom, don't turn on the overhead or bedside light; instead, use a nightlight or flashlight to guide the way. Interestingly, on the flip side, you should make sure to get plenty of natural light during the day, which is important for melatonin regulation.

◆ **No-tech, no-work zone**: Leave your electronic work and communication devices outside the bedroom door; the glow they give off can be disruptive to sleep. Cover your digital clock, as well as anything else that emits light, with a thick towel. If you have a computer or television in your bedroom, which isn't recommended, shut them off or cover them as well. Also, make sure you never work or study in your bed; condition your brain to relax in bed, not spin on work-related topics.

- **Exercise early**: For some, exercising within three hours of bedtime can disrupt sleep, as the levels of cortisol in the body are still high, acting to keep the brain alert, so mornings and afternoons are best for exercise if you want to get a good night's sleep.[144]

- **Turn your brain off from your day:** Often it's hard for us to make our brain stop spinning at night, so try incorporating something into your routine that you know relaxes you. As mentioned earlier this could be reading, meditation, or even sex. Sex releases endorphins and oxytocin, both of which can help by reducing anxiety and promoting relaxation.[145]

- **Napping:** A short nap (twenty to thirty minutes) is recommended to improve short-term alertness. This type of nap improves performance but doesn't leave you feeling groggy and will not interfere with nighttime sleep.[146]

- **Worry list:** Before you go to bed, try writing down the things you need to get done the next day or things you are worried about. By writing them down, you get them out of your head.

- **Relax:** An hour before bedtime, try to mediate, use guided imagery, listen to music, practice yoga breathing, or read. Avoid things like balancing your checkbook or watching violent television shows or movies. You can condition yourself to fall asleep to guided imagery. In fact, after a while, you will be able to fall asleep after only hearing the first few minutes or so.

- **Food and drink:** Drinking alcohol at or after dinner may help you fall asleep quickly, but it is also likely to cause you to wake up several hours later. Also skip caffeine for about five to seven hours directly before bed. It's probably also a good idea to stay away from nicotine, highly sugared desserts, chocolate, and big meals at dinner or after midafternoon. Chamomile or lavender teas are good ways to relieve some stress, soothe your mind and body, and help you sleep.

Are you getting enough sleep? Do you feel rested most mornings? Take the time to write down three to five things you will try to improve your sleep:

Sometimes it helps to track your sleep to see how it changes and determine what things affect it. A variety of sleep monitors and sleep apps on the market can provide you with good feedback. Some fitness trackers also have sleep-monitoring functions. Personally, I am not a fan of these because it is better to keep technology away from your bedroom.

If your insomnia lasts for weeks or months even after trying all the suggestions mentioned here, you should go see your primary care physician. He or she can help to assess the reasons you are not sleeping and provide additional guidance on sleep-inducing remedies (melatonin, acupuncture, and so on). The point is to just make sure you are consciously prioritizing a good night's sleep and forming a routine that works best for you and allows you to get at least seven hours of sleep. It will truly help with all other aspects of your health!

✅ TAKE CHARGE OF YOUR HEALTH

1. Do an assessment of your bedroom. Is it peaceful, calm, and promoting good sleep? If not, think about the changes that you can make to improve your surroundings and then incorporate them.

2. Try for two weeks to go to bed at the same time every night and wake up at the same time the next morning.

3. Before you go to bed, jot your worries down in a journal or in an app to get them out of your head and help you sleep more peacefully.

4. If possible, eliminate cell phones, computers, and so forth, from your bedroom.

4

Making Time for Your Mental and Emotional Health

 n the next subject area, you will learn about the connection between mental/emotional health and your
overall well-being. Three specific areas will be discussed in
the next sections: understanding mental health, finding your
passion in life, and connecting with your sexual health.

PRIORITIZING YOUR MENTAL HEALTH

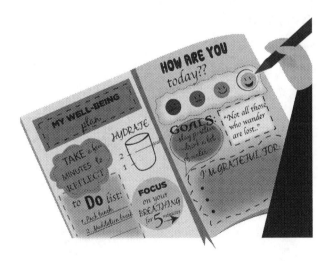

This is an extremely important topic to me because as I
have seen (and experienced) for decades, there is always

a clear connection between physical health and mental well-being. The two must be synchronized. However, mental health is often a comparatively tough area to talk about. Compare it to a broken arm or leg. You can see broken limbs, but you cannot see a broken heart or mind; only the people suffering can see their own pain. There is also still so much stigma in this arena, but it's important to remember that we can all help to change that with acceptance and love, both for ourselves and for others. As mentioned earlier, at age twenty-one, I had to make a painful and extremely personal choice: to continue living or not. I am so thankful for reaching out for help; this decision changed my life. I hope this chapter can teach you how to understand the importance of mental well-being and key components and get help if you need someone to lean on.

FACTS YOU NEED TO KNOW

1. One in five women in the US experienced a mental health condition in the past year.[147]

2. Routine stress, or stress related to work and family, can contribute to mental health disorders such as depression and anxiety.[148]

1. Only 50 percent of adults with mental health problems receive treatment.[149]

2. Premenstrual Syndrome (PMS) affects 30 to 80 percent of women, with symptoms such as anxiety, depression, anger, irritability, and social withdrawal.[150]

3. An average of one in nine new mothers will experience postpartum depression, and this can be as high as one in five depending on the state.[151]

ESSENTIAL INFO

What caused this mental health challenge? There are so many expectations placed on women today. We are expected to take care of our families, be terrific volunteers in the community and at the kids' schools, and have fabulous careers, all while staying fit, beautiful, and sexy. With that kind of pressure, is it any wonder women suffer from both anxiety and depression?

Too often, we as women put our time, energy, and efforts into helping others, neglecting to pay attention to our own needs. However, for the sake of your mental well-being, you must take the time to take care of yourself.

The good news is there are actions you can take in your everyday life to combat this pressure and improve your mental well-being. You cannot always change a stressful situation, but you are in control of the way you react to it. It is crucial to recognize when things aren't going well in this arena. Your body will send you many clues; you may notice pains, tiredness, headaches, and so forth, when you aren't in a good mental place. However, we often ignore these clues! Listen to what your body is telling you.

Think about your behavior as well. Are you usually a person who runs on time but nowadays you are always late? Or are you usually someone who gets energy from socializing but right now you don't want to be around anyone? Try to make these observations honestly and without self-blame. The goal here is simply to stop and assess your current emotional/mental health so that you can improve it where and however possible.

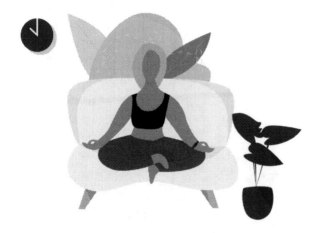

It is not helpful for you to feel overwhelmed. Recognize where your limits are and when you have reached them; know when it is time to pull back.[152] If, when you look at the state of your mental well-being, you realize that it's not where you want it to be, there are many healthy options you can try to help yourself. Here are some tips:

1. Pause! Take a break and do something else: take a deep breath, call a friend, go for a walk, or do any type of enjoyable activity that will help you come back into balance.[153]

2. It may sound counterintuitive, but you can also try altering your diet. Research suggests that a well-balanced diet with a high intake of whole grains, leafy vegetables, and fruit can reduce the risk of depression.[154]

3. You may want to think about how you can work physical activity into your schedule; it doesn't have to be strenuous to reap the benefits. Getting at least thirty minutes of exercise three to five days per week may significantly improve symptoms of depression and

anxiety. Half an hour of walking every day is a great way to rebalance your energy, bring up your energy level if you are depressed, or dissipate some excess energy if you are anxious.[155]

4. Another skill that I find to be particularly important and helpful for women is the ability to say no to things you really don't want to do. Don't put yourself into the black hole of remorse ... Life is short, and every moment matters. Try to spend your time the way you want. Pay attention to how you feel when the phone rings and you see who it is or how you feel before meeting someone for lunch. You need to be having this information loop with your mind, body, psyche, and spirit. If you start feeling anxious or you are dreading the encounter, then you need to look at the relationship and see what it is costing you in terms of your mental well-being. Focus on what you feel and act accordingly. I love the saying that if when asked to do something, your response isn't "hell yes," then the answer should be "no."

5. Practice mindfulness. Be mindful. Be here now. It is easy these days to get distracted with all our responsibilities and technological advances. Mindful meditation helps build the gentle perspective of self-observation without judgment, which can help improve your mental well-being in all aspects of your life.

6. Try guided imagery. If you can't make the time to learn to meditate and want something that will help you relax quickly, try guided imagery. With this as well, there are apps and audios on the market where all you need to do is press PLAY. The experience is sort of like a guided daydream. The words, tone of voice,

pacing, and background music will transport you into a relaxed, immersive, altered state. The pacing will tell your primitive brain that it is okay to relax and that things are safe. Then a voice will walk you through multisensory ideas, images, places, and themes that are going to occupy your brain and nourish it by giving it a break from stress and anxiety. Because guided imagery is so deeply relaxing, you come back from one of these imaginary trips feeling refreshed. Even if you fall asleep, you will wake up in much better shape! Fortunately, you don't need any training and it does not take learned discipline.

Getting started is easy with the help of all the resources available through today's technology; you can practice mindfulness, relaxation, and guided imagery right on your cell phone. For some of my absolute favorite resources, please see "Appendix 5—Helpful Mental Well-Being Resources."

Ask for help! There is no shame in admitting you need help so don't be afraid to ask for it. If possible, speak to a trusted family member or friend. If you know you need help but aren't sure where to turn, contact your employer's human resources or benefits department to find out about the resources available to you through your medical benefits or the employee assistance program. If you don't have health insurance, you will have to pay for services out of your own pocket or you can tap into some other resources that are available at low or no cost. See "Appendix 6—Low- or No-Cost Health Resources."

> Are you feeling overwhelmed or finding it hard to balance all your stressors? In thinking about your own current life, please take the time to write one to two new ways you will try to improve your mental well-being.

☑ TAKE CHARGE OF YOUR HEALTH

1. Set aside fifteen minutes a day (to start) as time for yourself. During that time, do whatever you want. When this becomes a habit, add more time.

2. Start practicing saying no to things you don't want to do.

3. Listen to a guided imagery audiotape or meditate each day (or when you can) and start with just five minutes! Health Journeys have donated a Take 5 series. Go to this link to start your Take 5 session: https://www.healthjourneys.com/prioritizing-yourself.

And of course remember to celebrate the little wins as you make these mental health changes—if you take three steps forward and one step back, you are still two steps ahead! More time for self-care is a big win so don't be too hard on yourself if you are having trouble remembering to prioritize yourself at first; life changes are not always comfortable and take time to become the new healthy habit.

FINDING YOUR PASSION

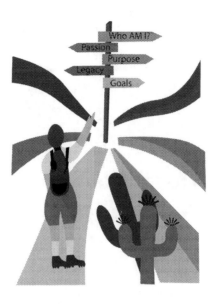

As I well know, when you get a second chance at life through a life-changing event or hitting rock bottom, you realize life is short. Each day, hour, and second is important and precious. Not everyone thinks about this when they wake up, but you may want to start. Living with passion and purpose gives life focus and clarity and can help improve all aspects of your health. For example, a greater sense of purpose has been associated with a greater use of preventive health care and fewer hospitalizations. Additionally, there is evidence to suggest that purpose in life is directly related to improved mental health and better coping skills when it comes to recovering from physical injuries or surgeries.[156] It's also important to remember that this purpose or passion is not one massive achievement on which you can hang your hat; it's a focus in life that allows you to feel like you are living your days well and contributing to something (or multiple things) bigger than yourself. Often, however, a lack of desire to live with purpose is what keeps us from being able to do it;

it's simply the fact that we have not yet discovered our passion. Maybe you are constantly checking things off your list, which feels good, but are you really enjoying the process? Enjoying the journey? So many of us aren't, so maybe that should be our new focus, our new challenge to ourselves. How do we design our lives in a way that allows us to truly enjoy the process of living, not just checking the boxes? It sounds great, so I hope you can use this chapter to help you give it a shot.

FACTS YOU NEED TO KNOW

1. Research suggests that living with purpose can improve cognitive function and protect against Alzheimer's disease.[157]

2. Having a sense of purpose has been linked to reduced stress, improved coping, and health-promoting behaviors.[158, 159]

3. A greater sense of purpose in life has been associated with a 50 percent reduction in the likelihood of stroke.[160, 161]

4. Studies show that people reporting a greater sense of purpose lived longer than their counterparts did. A sense of purpose has been shown to lower the risk of death by all causes by 15 percent.[162]

5. Evidence suggests that a greater sense of purpose in life can predict a higher household income.[163]

6. Having a sense of purpose can lead to positive emotions and reduce the likelihood of experiencing symptoms of depression.[164]

7. Research shows that living purposefully is associated with better quality sleep and a reduction in symptoms of insomnia.[165]

⚙ ESSENTIAL INFO

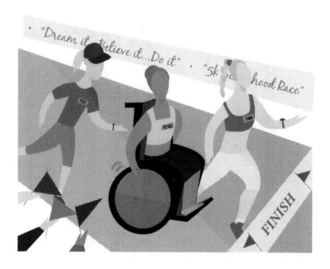

What is your purpose in life? So how do you identify *your* purpose in life so that you can start living it? The first step to finding your purpose is to determine the answer to the question "Who am I?" As a helpful prompt, try thinking of some of the times in your life when you were most excited, passionate, and productive. Answer the following questions about those times:

1. What were you doing?
2. Who were you with?
3. Where were you?
4. When were you doing it?
5. Why were you doing it?

Then list times in your life when you had no passion or sense of accomplishment and ask yourself the same five questions. Spend time analyzing the information you have written down and look for common themes. What did you learn about yourself and what motivates you and gives you a sense of passion?

Have You Thought about Your Personality Type?

If you want to learn even more about yourself and you haven't already done so, I highly recommend taking one (or more) of these personality assessments. Success in life and in your career is often tied to a deeper understanding of your personality and an authentic, positive, and purposeful application of that knowledge.

Personality assessments are a great tool to help you get there because they not only help you discover and analyze the characteristics that make you unique but also help you see yourself in an objective manner. For example, personality assessments will help you identify your strengths and give you information on how you tend to interact with others, your communication style, how others may perceive you, how you build relationships, how you listen, how you handle conflict, how you approach challenges, how you tend to lead others, and so forth. This information can then be used to create a more comprehensive and deeper level of self-awareness, which has been directly correlated with success, personal fulfillment, and the ability to have a greater, more positive influence on others. In addition, the assessments are often free, so there is really no downside!

For a simpler assessment (and free online), you can try The 5 Love Languages[166] or the Color Code Personality Test.[167] These are easy to take and the results can be eye-openers for you!

However, you may want to take an even more in-depth assessment that provides more comprehensive and formally usable information; look for ones that are often administered by certified professionals. Check with your company's human resources department to see if there are any available resources through work.

These detailed assessments will typically include a mapping of your personality style on a grid, information on your personality traits, where you fall in relation to norms in the general population, and career fit suggestions. Some assessments will even identify what you need from your environment to "be your best" and give you advice on how best to deal with stress in various situations. Please see "Appendix 7—Personality Assessments." By completing one or more of these assessments, you will likely gain some additional objective insights about yourself and the type of career that may help you find purpose in life.

Legacy and Purpose—What Does This Mean?

A friend shared a wonderful poem with me: "The Dash," by Linda Ellis.[168] The poem helps the reader reflect on the inherent value of living your life in a way you feel is worthwhile. It highlights the importance of what we do in between being born and dying. The dash is the in-between part of your life, what I call your "legacy."

Your personal legacy is your declaration of how you'd like to live your life and affect others. It is not about your goals or specific achievements but is meant to clearly set out your principles, how you intend to treat others, how you plan to care for yourself, and how you will share your legacy. This concrete approach will help give you focus and keep you on track as you deal with everyday challenges, also providing guidance for your mission in life and creation of your purpose statement.

Now that you have learned some of the benefits of discovering your purpose, begun to think about "Who Am I?", perhaps taken one of the free personality assessments or one of the more comprehensive assessments, and thought about the legacy you want to leave, it is time to create your purpose statement. Here are some examples of purpose statements for you to consider as you begin your journey and create your own:

- I want to be a recognized leader in health care and inspire women to be their best self.
- I want to lead by example and instill in my children the enormous value of being kind, honest, and having integrity.
- I want to grow in my profession successfully while staying committed to prioritizing myself.

Take the time to write your purpose statement below:

_____

_____

_____

_____

Once you think you know what your purpose might be, share and discuss themes with trusted friends, family members, or coworkers. What you are looking for is feedback, insights, and comments from people who know you. After you have talked through it with people who know you well, share your findings with a respected but neutral person, someone you do not consider a mentor or a friend, and see if you learn something new from their perspective.

It can be hard to live with purpose without support. Identify a mentor or accountability partner who can help you along the way. In addition, since we are constantly exposed to new information and situations, it is important to review and renew your purpose statement on an annual basis to make sure it still makes sense for you and reflects who you are.

Good luck, and enjoy finding and living up to your passion and purpose!

☑ TAKE CHARGE OF YOUR HEALTH

1. For one month, jot down what made you most happy and energized each day. Afterward, analyze these actions and feelings for any trends that might provide a window into your life's purpose.

2. Volunteer for sixty to ninety minutes or just talk with the leadership of a charity that you have long admired but have not "had the time" to do. Pay attention to how the experience affects your thoughts and feelings.

3. Write your purpose statement. Then think about whether or not you are currently contributing toward your desired legacy. Review it once a year to help you stay on track.

═══ **PAYING ATTENTION TO YOUR SEXUAL HEALTH** ═══

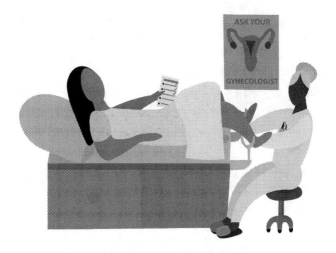

Although adding this part to my book raised some eyebrows from my advisory team, I felt it was essential for my audience to have a safe place to get guidance on some key sexual health issues. Did you know that if you search the words "sexual health," you will see over a billion results? There are many resources and places available to learn about ourselves, but often we fail to do so because, historically, talking about our sexual health or preferences was considered taboo. There are so many questions most of us never asked, such as the following: What is normal? What are the sexual parts of my body? What are they called? What is menstruation? Should I douche? How do I get pregnant? What do I do if I do? I want to have sex, but by the time I get to bed, all I can think about is sleeping—is this normal? Unless you grew up in a home where this was discussed and you were provided with the facts, you probably had to learn via trial and error. But using trial and error to learn about our own bodies is not only crazy; it's risky! You could end up with sexually transmitted diseases, unwanted pregnancies, and deep-seated shame. However, the good news is that it's never too late to learn. Let's try to overcome your discomfort at the taboo nature of this topic and really dive in and learn the answers to many of the questions you were never able to ask. There are many benefits of a fulfilling sex life that you should enjoy, including decreased stress and better sleep.[169]

 ## FACTS YOU SHOULD KNOW

1. Female sexual dysfunction, including desire, arousal, orgasm, or pain disorders, is a prevalent problem, affecting an estimated 43 percent of women.[170]

2. Psychological causes of sexual dysfunction include work-related stress and anxiety, concern about sexual performance, marital or relationship problems, depression, feelings of guilt, and the effects of past sexual trauma.[171]

3. One in four women has been raped by the time she turns forty-four years old.[172]

4. Condom use is rather uncommon—one in four acts of sexual intercourse are protected by a condom.[173]

5. The average adult has sex fifty-four times per year, lasting about thirty minutes.[174]

6. On average, the typical married person has sex fifty-one times per year; "very happy" couples have sex seventy-one times per year.[175]

ESSENTIAL INFO

Sexual health is a fundamental component of good health and has important implications for your overall health and quality of life.[176] There is nothing wrong with wanting a healthy and satisfying sex life! In fact, engaging in regular sexual activity is healthy because masturbation or sex with a partner helps keep the vagina properly stretched. While there is no denying the gender double standards when it comes to desiring sex, know that it is okay for you as a woman to want sex. Your sexuality should give you a sense of fulfillment and joy.

To get us started, let's talk about your period. What a fun topic, right? Your period is also called your "menstrual cycle" and is clinically defined as the hormonal process a woman's body goes through each month to prepare for a possible pregnancy.[177] I define it as the most important time of the month to take really good care of yourself—mentally and physically.

Regular menstrual periods in the years between puberty and menopause are usually a sign that your body is working normally. Irregular or heavy, painful periods should *not* be considered normal.[178] The menstrual cycle is typically counted from the first day of one period to the first day of the next period. The cycle may occur every twenty-one to thirty-five days, depending on the woman, and lasts from two to seven days on average.[179]

It's probably hard to remember off the top of your head when your last period was, how long it lasted, or if it was heavy or painful, so I highly recommend tracking your cycles. This can help you understand what is normal for you and help you identify important changes in your health should they occur, like a missed period or bleeding in between. Keep in mind that it doesn't mean something is "wrong" just because something changes, but being aware of your normal as well as unusual occurrences will make it easy for you to keep your doctor up to date so he or she can let you know if something is concerning.

Tracking your cycle with an app is super convenient and helps collect helpful information for you to track periods efficiently and accurately. In "Appendix 8—Apps for Tracking Your Periods," you will find some of my favorites.

You may be wondering when changes are serious enough to alert your doctor. If you have any of these symptoms, it would be worth a phone call to your gynecologist:[180]

1. Your period cycle changes
2. Your periods stop for more than ninety days (without a pregnancy)
3. Your period occurs more often than every twenty-one days or less often than every thirty-five days
4. Your bleeding continues for more than seven days
5. You bleed between periods
6. You experience extremely painful periods
7. You develop a fever and feel ill after using tampons
8. Your bleeding is heavier than usual or you are soaking through one pad or tampon every one to two hours

As we all know, even when things are going normally, being on your period can be a drag. Here are some suggestions to help you manage your periods more effectively:

1. Always be prepared. Have your *unscented* tampons or pads easily available (at home, in your car, at work, in your book bag/briefcase/purse).
2. Always wash your hands before (and after) changing tampons.
3. Make sure your partner is aware of your cycle so they can be informed and supportive.

4. Don't wear tight-fitting clothes—wear your more comfortable clothes in case you feel bloated.
5. Keep your exercise lighter, focusing on activities like walking or yoga.
6. Drink plenty of water.
7. Make healthful food choices to improve your stamina.
8. Avoid consuming caffeine to ease the edginess.
9. Get enough sleep so your body can rejuvenate.
10. Use a hot water bottle to alleviate cramps.
11. Be extra kind to yourself.

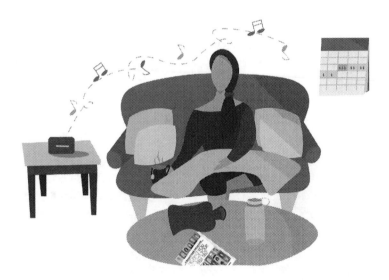

As part of taking care of your sexual health, it is very important to understand your anatomy. Too often, this is treated as taboo and overlooked, but understanding the scientific names of your anatomy is a critical element so you can speak with your physician about health concerns or pain using the correct terminology.

The Anatomy of Your Vulva

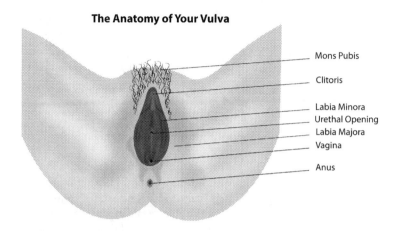

Mons Pubis

Clitoris

Labia Minora
Urethal Opening
Labia Majora
Vagina

Anus

For the purposes of this workbook, I am not going into details on all aspects of sex. But as you think about your own anatomy and your own sex life, you might be wondering what is "normal." I think two topics are extremely important to acknowledge with respect to normalcy: first, orgasms by penetration, and second, vaginal odor.

Regarding the first point, most women think there is something wrong with them if they are not reliably orgasmic with penetration. The reality is that the *majority of women* are not reliably orgasmic with penetration. This is because the clitoris is the most sensitive sex organ for women and is not internal to the vagina. About half of women sometimes have orgasms with intercourse, which is because they have nerve endings in their vaginas that are more sensitive than other women's are.[181] Don't feel abnormal if you cannot orgasm that way; remember, you are in the majority!

Second, women often believe their vaginas have an unpleasant odor and turn to douching. Douching is actually more harmful than it is helpful. It is a myth that douching makes you cleaner. In reality, douching strips away good bacteria and leaves you more vulnerable to bacterial and yeast infections. If you have an existing infection when you douche, the bacteria can get pushed to your reproductive organs, causing pelvic inflammatory disease, which could also lead to fertility problems.[182] Are these enough reasons not to douche? There is no need to be uncomfortable with your natural scent, but if you notice a change in scent, or discharge and an odor, have a discussion with your gynecologist.

Sexual Dysfunctions—The Two You Should Know

Let's talk a little more about what can go wrong with your sexual health. Primarily, it's important to note that sexual problems are incredibly common in adult women of all ages. About 30 to 50 percent of women have sexual problems at some time during their lives.[183]

Two common sexual dysfunctions are hypoactive sexual desire disorder (HSDD) and the genitourinary syndrome of menopause (GSM).

1. HSDD is the most prevalent sexual condition in women of all ages. It is defined as the absence of or persistent decrease in sexual interest, including sexual thoughts, dreams, fantasies, response, and desire, and it often causes personal distress.[184] HSDD can be brought on by mental stressors and has immense negative impacts on women's overall health. For example, HSDD often negatively affects a woman's body image, causing a vicious cycle to ensue. Interestingly, in this case, it is typically not the body image that affects the sex drive; rather, having poor sexual function often negatively impacts a woman's body image, perception of self-worth, self-confidence, and sense of connectedness with her partner, in turn further depleting her sexual desires.[185]

2. GSM is a result of the loss of estrogen at menopause, which impacts more than 50 percent of postmenopausal women. Symptoms include dryness, burning or irritation in the genitals, poor vaginal lubrication during sex, and an urgent need to urinate.[186] The term GSM was developed in 2014 as a result of a consensus conference of menopause and sexual health experts. It was important to develop a new term because while GSM includes vulva vaginal atrophy (VVA), many media outlets prohibit the use of the anatomically correct term vagina, so there is no public awareness for treatment of VVA.[187] Additionally, vaginal atrophy only refers to the vagina, but when you lose estrogen, it affects other parts of the urogenital tract as well, such as the bladder. Because it takes time for that loss of estrogen to have an impact, GSM often starts a bit later than menopause, meaning women often don't realize the direct cause and effect. This means they also often fail to realize that there are safe and effective treatments for it.[188]

The Biopsychosocial Side of Sex

The best way to understand sexual concerns is to recognize that they involve many variables. Biology, psychology and the way you were socialized all impact your sexual thought process. That means you need to consider all the components that contribute to healthy and functioning sexual health in order to fully understand and alleviate your concerns.

On the biological side, we know that hormones, brain chemistry, physical health, and having a chronic disease or condition all impact sexual health. In fact, desire itself has biological components: neurotransmitters. For example, dopamine is an important neurotransmitter for sexual reward processing, excitement, and sexual pleasure.[189] Serotonin, which has a positive impact on mood, is not great for sex drive. The balance of those neurotransmitters can have a healthy or dysfunctional impact.[190]

On the psychological side, suffering from anxiety, depression, or other issues can interfere with healthy sexual function. Your mental well-being matters and therefore needs to be considered as being part of your sexual health too.[191] If you are struggling and feel that your mental health or thoughts are affecting your sexual drive, get help.

Sociocultural factors, which also include religious and cultural beliefs, also have a huge impact on women's sexual health. Finally, interpersonal factors like the quality of the relationship have a major impact on healthy sexual function.[192] Let's think about what that means. You could have all the biological drive in the world, but if you don't like or trust your partner, you are not going to want to be sexual. On the other hand, you could have a great relationship, but if biologically your neurotransmitters are off balance, then the ability to process reward and to have sexual interest is not going to be there. If you are concerned about your sexual well-being or you are experiencing issues, you need to think about all of these components and determine which need to be addressed.

Making Time for Sex

A common challenge for many of us is finding the time for sex. If you are overwhelmed with work, family, or both and are exhausted by nightfall, the last thing you may be thinking about is making love with your partner. To that, I say *please* rethink this notion because the connection you will feel with the person you love is priceless and worth the effort and time spent for you both. The sexual aspects of a loving relationship are a great way to stay connected on a truly intimate level. In the fitness discussion, I suggested making an appointment for your exercise time and keeping it. Now I would like you to consider making time for sex by putting it on the calendar as an event! **Note: You may want to have a secret way of blocking the time off the calendar so that everyone who has access to your calendar is not aware of the specifics of this appointment.** Scheduling time for sex during the week may seem a bit mechanical, but I also think it adds to the foreplay as both partners look forward to their special "date time." You can even take turns planning your time together. Speak openly with your partner to see if they are willing to try this with you.

It's Fun to Be Creative

You may want to also consider being creative in the bedroom—sex toys can help. Research shows that about 53 percent of US women use a vibrator,[193] and it's totally okay to bring the vibrator into the bedroom for use with a partner! Many American couples use sex toys during sexual activity to add a little spice and fun.

Do remember, though, to be very careful to wash them thoroughly before and after use and never to switch over a toy from the anus to the vagina without washing it. Toys made from porous materials tend to trap bacteria and cannot be completely disinfected. To remedy this, use a condom over the toy to add protection. For nonporous toys such as hard plastic, elastomer, metal, glass, or silicone, be sure to wash with a mild disinfecting, nonirritating soap and water before and after each use.

Sexually Transmitted Infections

It is also important to acknowledge that sexual activity with nonpermanent partners carries a higher risk of contracting a sexually transmitted infection. Here are some stats for you to consider:

1. One in two sexually active persons will contract a sexually transmitted infection (STI) by age twenty-five.[194]

2. It is estimated that 24,000 women become infertile each year due to undiagnosed STIs.[195]

3. Researchers estimate that at least 80 percent of sexually active people will have a human papillomavirus (HPV) infection at some point in their lifetime. HPV is responsible for approximately 31,500 cases of cancer each year, including nearly all cases of cervical and anal cancer, about 75 percent of vaginal cancer, 70 percent of oropharyngeal cancer, and 69 percent of vulvar cancer.[196]

4. Herpes infection is common. About one in eight people aged fourteen to forty-nine in the US has genital herpes.[197]

If you are sexually active outside of a long-term monogamous relationship, regardless of your age, make sure to practice safe sex. Also, before anyone starts touching you, make sure they have washed their hands. That might not sound very sexy, but it's extremely important to ensure that hands that have touched all kinds of bacteria have been freshly cleaned before they touch you—outside and inside.

Additionally, condoms are the best choice for penetrative sex, including the use of a condom on a dildo. Older women may think they don't need to use one since they aren't worried about pregnancy, but the fact is that older women are even *more* at risk for infection as the tissue becomes more fragile and gets thinner, increasing the risk for sexually transmitted infections.[198]

Also, always bear in mind that infections can be transmitted via oral sex as well, so talk to your partner. Ask about getting tested and when his/her last test was.

Final Thoughts to Consider

1. If your health-care provider is not asking you about sexual health during your annual exams, find a clinician who will. Or bring up the topics yourself by saying something like, "I have some questions and concerns about my sexual health." Categories include desire, arousal, ability to reach orgasm, and any pain with sexual activity. Remember, you have every right to be asking about sexual health and should not feel embarrassed or as if you are being inappropriate by bringing it up.

2. Two other great topics to stay in touch with your physician about are contraception and menopause. Each of these topics could be their own entire workbook, so make sure to keep these in mind and talk openly with your doctors about them.

    ♦ As a quick overview, birth control (contraception) is any method, medicine, or device used to prevent pregnancy. Many are over the counter, while some require prescriptions. Some work better than others do at preventing pregnancy. The type of birth control you use depends on your health, your desire to have children now or in the future, and your need to prevent sexually transmitted diseases. It is important to think about what works best for you and your lifestyle. Take the time to investigate and have a thoughtful discussion with your doctor and your partner. But do always remember that as women, the ultimate responsibility for birth control sits with us. Therefore, it is your responsibility to start the discussions and find and stick to a method that works for you.

◆ The absence of menstrual periods for twelve-plus months is called menopause. During this time, your ovaries cease to function. The average age of women experiencing menopause is fifty-one years old but varies and can range from the thirties to the sixties.[199] It is important to track your menstrual cycles so that you can notice any variance from normal. Some women go through menopause with few symptoms; others may experience a variety of symptoms (I experienced most of these), including hot flashes, weight gain, mood swings, acne, changes in skin texture, incontinence, memory problems, night sweats, painful intercourse, and vaginal and urinary problems. It is very important to discuss your symptoms with your doctor and come up with the best plan to support your transition. **Important note: If you have any spotting once you are in menopause, you must immediately contact your doctor for advice and follow-up; this could be a symptom of cancer and needs to be evaluated.**[200]

I am hoping by now that you will not let embarrassment get in the way of taking care of your sexual health and that you have learned the importance of this aspect of your health. Know that your gynecologist is equipped with the answers you need to know.

☑ TAKE CHARGE OF YOUR HEALTH

1. Practice using sexual terminology. Write down questions that you might otherwise be embarrassed or uncomfortable asking your gynecologist. Take the questions with you when you go see your doctor and be sure to ask them.

2. Ask your doctor to use a mirror when you are having a pelvic exam so that when a speculum is inserted, you can see what your vagina looks like and maybe even get a glimpse of your cervix. Remember that it is your body and there is no need to feel embarrassed!

3. Sit in front of a mirror and spread your legs to see what your labia inner lips and outer lips look like, where your clitoris is, where your vaginal opening is, and what your vulva looks like. Do you know your anatomy?

5

Navigating Your
Financial Health

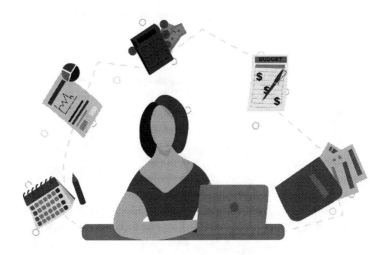

*F*inancial health is the last part of well-being that will be covered in this guide. If you have your finances in sync, with revenue meeting or exceeding expenses, it can greatly reduce your stress and improve your overall health and happiness.

> I had to include a chapter on financial health because it has been such an integral part of my health journey, being that I have been making my own way since I was seventeen years old. So many of us rack up an

extraordinary amount of debt and then are left with no idea of how to overcome it. This is just the result of a lacking underlying under-standing about how to parse our income ver-sus our expenses. When we think about how to take care of ourselves, financial education is often deprioritized because it's difficult (and, let's face it, often boring). However, trying to get out of debt is extremely stressful and can wreak havoc on our health as well as nega-tively impact our families and our relationships. Remember that having a better understand-ing of your financials will contribute materially to overall wellness and protect you during the phases of your life.

FACTS YOU NEED TO KNOW

1. The average gender pay gap in the US is around 19.3 percent, meaning that a woman working a full-time year-round job earns 81.6 percent as much as her male counterpart earns. That gap can be larger or smaller, depending on the state someone lives in.[201]

2. Two-thirds (66.2 percent) of working millennials have nothing saved for retirement. This situation is far worse for working millennial Latinos, as 83 percent have nothing saved for retirement.[202]

3. Of all women sixty-five and over, 16 percent are living at or below poverty levels.[203]

4. Stress resulting from financial challenges is often chronic—affecting 26 percent of Americans most or all of the time.[204]

⚙ ESSENTIAL INFO

If you don't have any idea how retirement planning works, you're not alone. Many women are embarrassed to admit that they don't know much about planning for retirement or that they haven't even given it much thought. Yet over half of all women in the US today are single and living alone and may retire without a partner.[205] Regardless of whether we are single, married, divorced, or in a committed relationship, we should have our own retirement plans and accounts. Women can handle their finances just as skillfully as the stereotypical man can—we just need to know what to do and not do and have the confidence to get it done. So where do you start?

Primarily, you need to look at your finances now. How much are you spending each month on the necessities versus the nonessentials, or discretionary spending? Necessities include your living expenses, such as your mortgage or rent, utilities, automobile expenses, groceries, debt payments, medical expenses, savings, retirement contributions, and taxes.

Incidental discretionary spending includes things like a gym membership, haircut and color, gifts for holidays, vacations, or major shopping sprees. Day-to-day discretionary spending includes things like eating out, entertainment, books and magazines, makeup, a mani-pedi, and so forth. None of these discretionary purchases are a necessity, so you may be able to cut back or eliminate them from your monthly spending entirely if needed.

Once you have an idea of your monthly spending and how it breaks down, you can start to think about how to improve your current financial status if necessary. Cutting spending and eliminating debt are two great places to start.

Next you need to ask yourself some important questions before you begin retirement planning. What are your goals and objectives for the future? Are you saving to buy a car, house, or boat? Do you want to pay off student loans or credit cards? Do you want to save for your own retirement or for your children to go to college? Answering these questions will help you determine how to structure your savings plan.

The next step is to learn about the various types of investments available to determine which align best with your savings goals and choose an amount or percentage of your income to set aside each month or from each paycheck. You can adjust this at any time.

Important note: If all of this feels too overwhelming to take on yourself, or you would like a little more guidance than I provide here, contact a financial planner or advisor. Share your goals and discuss with them the best strategies for reaching those goals.

As part of the process of thinking about how much you want to set aside for the future, you also need to think about how much debt you have now. Consider the following:

1. Debt is the largest roadblock to establishing your retirement planning.

2. Forbes reports that student loan debt in the US averages $37,172 per borrower (for the class of 2016).[206]

3. Forty-one percent of Americans carry credit card debt, meaning that they can't meet their basic expenses without borrowing regularly at an average interest rate of 17 percent.[207]

Compounding interest on credit cards can be staggering. Let's say you make a $1,000 purchase using your credit card. The interest rate is 18 percent and your monthly minimum payment is 2.5 percent, or $25. If you only make the minimum payment each month, that $1,000 purchase will ultimately cost you $2,115.41, more than double its original price—not to mention that it will take you twelve years to pay off that amount if you continue to pay just the minimum payment. As a rule of thumb, you should never charge more to your credit card than you can afford to pay off completely.

What about Debt?

When you think about debt, always remember that there is *productive debt* and *unproductive debt*. Productive debt is money borrowed to finance an asset or productive activity that is expected to provide benefits over time. Examples are a mortgage or student loan. Unproductive debt, however, is money borrowed that is not to finance an asset, such as credit card debt or a long-term car loan, since a car will depreciate over time, not appreciate. Start by reducing and eliminating your highest cost unproductive debts and then pay down your productive ones.

You may be trying to decide whether it's better to save money or to pay down your debt. Let's say your credit card has an interest rate of 18 percent. The question you should ask yourself, then, is can you find an investment that has an 18 percent annual return with zero risk? Presumably, you cannot, which is why, before funding a retirement plan and before building a cash reserve, you need to pay off your credit card balances. Every dollar of principal reduction provides you a guaranteed financial return equal to the interest rate on your card. The higher the rate, the greater the guaranteed return. Investments in assets like stocks and bonds are anything but guaranteed, and a diversified mutual fund will rarely produce gains as generous as the rate you are paying to your bank for the privilege of using its credit card.

After looking at your long-term goals and paying down your unproductive debt, decide how to allocate your savings amongst different retirement accounts. Note that this can be confusing because of the many types of accounts available today. Retirement accounts are intended for *long-term tax-advantaged* savings accumulation and income security. There are rules for how much you can contribute to each type of plan, as well as rules for how much of your contribution you can deduct for income taxes. Each year, the IRS adjusts the contribution limits for inflation, which is helpful. Tax advantages come with many conditions and operating rules, so it's good to understand at least the basics before committing your hard-earned money.

Now you may be wondering about social security, thinking that because you already paid into it, doesn't that mean you are covered for retirement? Social security benefits replace about 40 percent of your salary on average when you retire; however, they are not meant to be your sole income. The average monthly social security check is $1,130, which likely is nowhere near enough to cover your monthly expenses.[208] In fact, even the combination of a retirement account and social security benefits is probably not enough. You will need additional savings to cover other unexpected expenses. Here are some examples that may seem like stretch goals but are definitely worth working to achieve:

1. **Regular Savings Account:** Your goal should be to have at least eight months' worth of expenses in a savings account.

2. **Emergency Savings Account:** This is a separate account where you reserve money for emergencies

that may occur. A serious illness or loss of income can wipe out your savings and leave you with nothing, so it's good to have a backup plan.

3. **Health Savings Account:** A health savings account, or HSA, is a tax-advantaged account that is paired with a high-deductible health plan. An HSA is intended for current or future health-care expenses that are not covered by insurance, such as deductibles and other out-of-pocket costs. Before age sixty-five, HSA funds you spend on anything but medical expenses are subject to income tax and a 20 percent penalty. At age sixty-five, contributions to the account must cease. The remaining funds are tax-free if spent for medical purposes. If spent for any other purpose, they are subject to tax but not to the 20 percent penalty.[209]

4. **College Savings Account:** Saving for college should start as soon as children are born. College savings accounts, such as 529 plans, work much like a Roth IRA by investing your after-tax contributions. The growth in the value of the account is completely tax-free as long as the funds are used for college tuition, room and board, books, and certain other qualified costs. Account earnings (not principal) used for any other purpose are subject to income tax plus a 10 percent penalty.[210]

5. **Dream Account:** If there are certain trips or goals you know you have for the future, save up in a special account until you can afford them! It's a far better approach than using a high-interest credit card to fund your excursions or experiences.

It can be a serious challenge to build up these tactical accounts, manage debt, and fund long-term retirement accounts. There is only so much money to go around! You shouldn't feel as if you have to tackle everything at once. Depending on your situation, the only practical way forward is to allocate your income and savings based on your personal judgment and priorities.

If you are still not sure exactly how you should be approaching all of this, look at some of my saving suggestions below, broken down by age. And of course remember that it's never too late (or too early!) to start saving for retirement.

Planning Your Finances through the Years

Financial goals change throughout our lifetimes, so I thought it would be helpful to provide a planning guide based on age ranges to assist you with your goals.

Twenties: Though you may not have a large salary, it is a great time to start saving for retirement to take advantage of compounding interest.

- Put at least 10 percent of your income in a retirement account and increase the amount you contribute by 1 percent each year until you reach 20 percent
- Create a budget and adopt a savings mentality
- Consider a Roth IRA account or Roth 401(k)
- Take charge of your student debt
- Be aggressive with your investments because you have time to make up for any losses

Thirties: If you haven't started saving for retirement by the time you are in your thirties, don't delay.

- Put at least 20 percent of your income in a retirement account

- Max out your 401(k) contribution
- Start building your non–retirement savings accounts to which you will contribute in your forties and fifties
- Pay down debt
- Consider investing in real estate by buying a home. Remember, this is an actual *investment*; it's not just about your "dream house"
- Continue to be aggressive with your investments because you still have plenty of time to make up for any losses

Forties: At this point, you need to be saving as much as you can for retirement.

- Examine your retirement account balance(s) and make adjustments if there is a shortfall
- Invest in lower-risk bonds, unless you have been neglecting your retirement savings plan
- Fine-tune your portfolio
- Pay off high-interest debt
- Set a clear retirement savings target
- Continue to be aggressive with your investments

Fifties: Retirement is getting close; you need to be ready.

- Make catch-up contributions to your tax-free savings plan
- Rebalance your portfolio
- Delay retirement if your retirement account is underfunded
- Get on a ten-year plan to debt freedom

Sixties: You're nearly there. Make sure everything is in order.

- By this time, you should be close to owning your home outright

- Don't be afraid to downsize
- Calculate how much longer you want to work
- Make sure all estate plans and documents are in order

Finally, I wanted to touch on some of the things you should *not* do when it comes to your financial future:

1. **Live on credit:** Consumer debt is like cancer. It starts small, but then it begins to grow. This kind of debt comes with high interest rates that can be hard to dig yourself out of.

2. **Live an overstated lifestyle:** Some people prefer the illusion of wealth and will spend every penny to keep up appearances. If your monthly extravagances keep you from preparing for retirement, you are living beyond your means.

3. **Strip home equity:** Many people turn to home equity loans or lines of credit to pay off high-interest credit card debt or simply to finance ordinary expenses. If you are unable to pay the steep mortgage payments each month, you'll end up losing your home through foreclosure.

4. **Raid retirement accounts:** Dipping into your retirement fund to pay off a credit card or cover some large home repair might seem like a good idea, but you will lose more than you gain. You will be charged a penalty—usually around 10 percent—for making a withdrawal before retirement age. Then you are required to pay back the loan amount to your retirement fund and could face additional taxes if you do not pay it back in the required time limit.

5. **Take out college loans:** I am referring to Parent Loans for Undergraduate Students (PLUS), not student loans. Repayment of these loans starts two months after the funds are received, and the total must be paid back in ten years. If you miss any payments, the loans grow monthly as the past-due amounts are added to the outstanding balance. It's better to take a student loan out on your own to avoid this situation.

6. **Procrastinate:** Many women assume it will be easier to save for retirement later in their careers because they will be more established. However, securing your financial future for retirement requires that you start saving now.

The bottom line is to focus on what savings you can start today and do the very best you can to build your retirement savings. Whatever amount you can contribute now is the right amount!

☑ TAKE CHARGE OF YOUR HEALTH

1. Create a budget that includes your income and expenses, monthly and annually, as well as set aside a portion for savings.

2. Transfer your budget information to a financial app that will allow you to monitor your spending.

3. Make an appointment with a certified financial advisor. *You may be able to connect through employer benefits or you can ask your friends for recommendations, though always be sure to check references.*

You've Got This!

Dear Sister of Our World,

As I said at the start of this guide, today is the first day of the rest of your life. Thank you so much for taking your time to let me share my thoughts and being open-minded about learning some ways to take better care of your health. You have a lot to think about as you continue your life journey and work toward ongoing health improvements. I hope that some of these chapters have encouraged you to think about yourself and some of the positive opportunities you have for changing your life for the better.

The changes I have suggested will take commitment, planning and practice in addition to taking time to achieve. Enjoy the process of change and try to celebrate each step along the way. Each small step is a win and will help you stick to realistic and sustainable goals overtime.

Love yourself as you love others. You are in control of your own destiny. You own your future and should know you've got this!

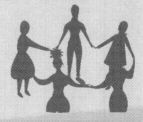

Healthfully yours,
Cheryl Agranovich

Appendixes

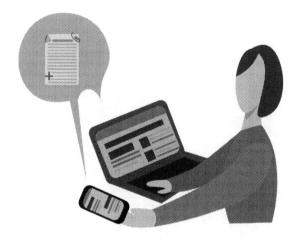

Appendix 1—Plant-based Resources

If you want to shift toward more plant-based proteins but you are not sure how to do so, wonderful resources are available:

Websites
- forksoverknives.com
- fruitsandveggies.org
- gamechangers.movie.com
- plantproof.com
- plantstrong.com
- pulses.org
- wholefoodplantbasedresources.com

Books
- *Eat to Live*, Joel Fuhrman, MD
- *Engine 2 Diet*, Rip Esselstyn
- *How Not to Die*, Michael Greger, MD, FACLM, with Gene Stone
- *How Not to Diet*, Michael Greger, MD, FACLM
- *The China Study Solution*, Thomas Colin Campbell, MD
- *The Forks Over Knives Plan*, Alona Pulde, MD and Matthew Lederman, MD
- *The Plant-based Journey*, Lani Mvelrath
- *The Vegan Starter Kit*, Neal Barnard, MD
- *Plant-Strong*, Rip Esselstyn
- *Whole: Rethinking the Science of Nutrition*, T. Colin Campbell

Films

- Diet Fiction
- Food Choices
- Forks Over Knives
- Gamechangers
- H.O.P.E. What You Eat Matters
- Live and Let Live
- Planeat
- Plant Pure Nation

Podcasts

- Nutrition Facts with Dr. Greger
- Rich Roll
- Plant Proof with Simon Hill
- Diet Fiction Podcast
- Engine 2 PlantStrong with Rip Esselstyn
- Food for Thought – Colleen Patrick-Goudreau

Appendix 2—Recipe Resources

New and easy recipes can make cooking fun and exciting. Here are some great resources for you as you expand your recipe collections (make your selections wisely):

Websites

- Allrecipes.com
- Chocolatecoveredkatie.com
- Cookieandkate.com
- Feastingonfruit.com
- Feastingathome.com
- Feelgoodfoodie.net
- Fitfoodiefinds.com
- Foodwithfeeling.com/category/vegan
- Forksoverknives.com/recipes
- Gamechangersmovie.com/food/recipes
- Itdoesnttastelikechicken.com
- Minimalistbaker.com
- Mydarlingvegan.com
- Noracooks.com
- Onegreenplanet.org
- Plantproof.com/category/recipes
- Skinnytaste.com
- Yummly.com

Slow Cooker Specific

- Countryliving.com
- Crock-pot.com
- Purewow.com
- Realhousemoms.com
- Sweetpeasand saffron.com
- Thepioneerwoman.com

Books

- *Forks Over Knives Flavor!,* Darshanna Thicker
- *Forks Over Knives The Cookbook,* Del Sroufe
- *How Not to Die Cookbook,* Michael Greger, MD
- *The China Study Cookbook,* Leanne Campbell, PhD
- *The Engine 2 Cookbook,* Rip Esselstyn and Jane Esselstyn
- *The No Meat Athlete Cookbook,* Matt Frazier and Stephanie Romine
- *Vegan Richa's Everyday Kitchen,* Richa Hingle

Appendix 3—Nutrition App Resources for You

Staying on track with your nutritional selections is made easy by using an app to ensure you are being accountable and getting all the necessary nutrients. Here are some of my favoite apps:

- LifeSum—Diet and Macro Tracker
- Lose It! Calorie Counter
- MyFitnessPal
- MyPlate Calorie Counter
- Noom
- Start Tracking

Appendix 4—Fitness App Resources for You

There are also several amazing fitness apps to help make fitness sustainability easy. Check out the ones below and find the best exercise program suited for you:

- Beachbody on Demand
- Blogilates
- Boxx Workout
- Peleton
- 7 Minute Workout by Wahoo Fitness
- 8 Fit Workout
- Jillian Michaels My Fitness Workout
- Map My Run
- Nike Training Club
- Shred
- Strava Workout
- Workout for Women
- YogaGlo

Appendix 5 - Mental Well-Being Resources

Tapping into mental well-being resources can help with managing stress and improve your overall health. Here are some of my favorites:

- **CALM** is an amazingly helpful meditation and relaxation aid. Geared toward supporting great sleep and improving performance, this program taps into technology to improve focus and reduce stress.
- **Happify** is your fast track to a good mood. This free app provides engaging games, activity suggestions, gratitude prompts and more to train your brain to overcome negative thoughts.
- **Headspace** provides guidance on everyday mindfulness and meditation for stress, anxiety, sleep, focus, fitness, and more.
- **Health Journeys** is a pioneer in this field. HJ features guided experiences by foremost experts in the mind-body field that address specific health and mental health conditions as well as ones that help people relax, de-stress, and sleep better. They feature an array of experts like Bodhipaksa (beautiful soothing voice), Tara Brach, Belleruth Naparstek, Jon Kabat-Zinn, and others.
- **Lifesum** is a broader resource for all things healthy living. The app allows you to set up personal goals that range from healthy eating to working out.
- **My3** is designed to help those stay safe while having thoughts of suicide. My3 is free and lets you customize your own personal safety plan by noting your warning signs, listing coping strategies, and connecting you to helpful resources to consult when you need them most.

- **Moodkit** uses the foundation of cognitive behavior therapy and provides users with more than 200 different mood improvement activities.
- **QuitThat** is a free habit tracker app that helps users beat their bad habits or addictions.
- **Ten Percent Happier** features Dan Harris as narrator, with nationally known mindful/meditation professionals such as Joseph Goldstein, Kelly McGonigal, Oren Jay Sofer, Sebene Selassie, Sharon Salzberg, and others. It offers guided meditations and practical advice for dealing with life in a fun and enlightening manner.

Appendix 6—Low- or No-Cost Mental Health Resources

If you don't have health insurance, you will either pay for services out of your own pocket or tap into other resources such as those listed here:

- **Your local health department:** Local health departments are designed to help protect, educate, and provide care within a community. These resources cover topics from flu shots to prenatal care.
- **United Way 2-1-1**: This program offers a comprehensive source for local human and social services support in the US and most of Canada. Support for crises, emergencies/disasters, food, health, human trafficking, housing/utilities, jobs/employment, reentry, and veterans.
- **Hospitals**: Many hospitals provide preventive care at low or no cost. Call your local hospital and ask what services they offer for people without health insurance. A good place to start is with the hospital's community resources department.
- **Planned Parenthood:** Planned Parenthood provides routine health-care services at low or no cost. Services may include (but are location-specific so check with your local Planned Parenthood office) anemia testing, testing for sexual health problems, cholesterol screening, colon cancer screening, diabetes screening, employment and sports physicals, flu vaccination, blood pressure screening, rape crisis counseling referrals, routine physical exams, smoking cessation programs, tetanus vaccination, thyroid screening, UTI testing and treatment, as well as other general services.

- **Medical schools:** Call a medical school in your area to inquire whether they provide any services to the community, including physicals, dermatology exams, eye, and dental checkups.
- **Other organizations:** Many organizations provide health screening services and education. Resources include the American Heart Association, American Diabetic Association, and the Red Cross, to name a few. These groups are nonprofits and are willing to provide help (at no charge) to those seeking additional support and education on a specific health issue.

Appendix 7—Personality Assessments

Personality assessments can improve how you communicate and relate to others. Examples of in-depth assessments include the following:

- **DISC Assessment:** Based on the ideas of psychologists William Marston and Walter Clarke, it evaluates behavior. It focuses on the traits of *dominance, inducement, submission, and compliance (DISC)*. Some companies rely on it to hire staff, while others use it to gauge an employee's suitability for a job. It may help put you on the career path that is right for you.
- **Process Communication Model:** The brainchild of NASA, this assessment groups people into six personality types. People are categorized as harmonizers, thinkers, rebels, imaginers, persisters, or promoters. Since this test assesses personal strengths, it may show you yours and help lead you to the perfect career.
- **The Birkman Method:** This tool measures a person's reaction to stress. It also considers strengths and social behavior.
- **The Enneagram:** This is a model of nine personality types: reformers, helpers, achievers, individualists, investigators, loyalists, enthusiasts, challengers, and peacemakers. It explains how the different personalities unite, also showing how nearby characters may influence each character.
- **The Myers-Briggs Type Indicator:** This is is one of the most popular personality assessment tests to date. It is based it on the ideas of psychoanalyst Carl Jung, who thought that people understood the world

through sensation, intuition, feeling, and thinking. While intuition and sensing help perception, feeling and thinking support judgment. The assessment also shows whether people are introverts or extroverts.

Appendix 8—Apps for Tracking Your Periods

Tracking your periods can provide valuable information for your health team. Here are some great tools available for you:

- Clue Period and Tracker
- Cycles Period and PMS Tracker
- Eve Period Tracker
- Flo Period and Ovulation Tracker
- Life
- Maya
- Menstrual Period Tracker
- Period Diary
- Period Tracker Lite

Notes

1   Paul D. Lopinzi, Adam Branscum, June Hanks, Ellen Smit, "Healthy Lifestyle Characteristics and Their Joint Association with Cardiovascular Disease Biomarkers in US Adults," *Mayo Clinic Proceedings* 91, no. 4 (April 2016): 432–442, https://doi.org/10.1016/j.mayocp.2016.01.009.

2   "About Chronic Diseases," National Center for Chronic Disease Control and Health Promotion, last reviewed October 23, 2019, https://www.cdc.gov/chronicdisease/about/index.htm.

3   "National Diabetes Statistics Report," Centers for Disease Control and Prevention, last reviewed February 24, 2018, https://www.cdc.gov/diabetes/data/statistics/statistics-report.html.

4   "Breast Cancer Risk in American Women," National Cancer Institute, last reviewed October 3, 2019, https://www.cancer.gov/types/breast/risk-fact-sheet.

5   Tim Newman, "The Numbers Behind Obesity," *Medical News Today*, October 27, 2017.

6   "Lower Your Risk for the Number 1 Killer of Women," Centers for Disease Control and Prevention Office of Women's Health, last reviewed February 7, 2018, https://www.cdc.gov/features/wearred/index.html.

7   Michael Gregor and Gene Stone, *How Not to Die: Discover the Foods Scientifically Proven to Prevent and Reverse Disease* (New York: Flatiron Books, 2015), 127.

8   Michael Gregor and Gene Stone, *How Not to Die*, 165.

9   Gretchen Borchelt, "The Impact Poverty Has on Women's Health," *American Bar Association Human Rights Magazine*, 43, no. 3, https://

www.americanbar.org/groups/crsj/publications/human rights magazine home/the-state-of-healthcare-in-the-united-states/poverty-on-womens-health/.

10 Joanne Finnegan, "Many Americans Don't Have a Primary Care Doctor," FierceHealthcare, accessed January 12, 2019, https://www.fiercehealthcare.com/practices/many-americans-don-t-have-a-primary-care-doctor.

11 Jack Ende, "Strengthening the Primary Care Workforce," National Coalition on Health Care Primary Care Forum, September 20, 2017, https://nchc.org/wp-content/uploads/2017/09/Jack-Ende.pdf.

12 Ende, "Strengthening the Primary Care Workforce."

13 Jaimie Dalessio Clayton, "Americans Research Cars More Closely Than Doctors," Everyday Health, last updated October 25, 2012, https://www.everydayhealth.com/healthy-living/1025/americans-research-cars-more-closely-than-doctors.aspx

14 Kristyna Wentz-Graff, "Women Responsible for Most Health Decisions in the Home," Oregon Health & Science University, May 11, 2017, https://news.ohsu.edu/2017/05/11/women-responsible-for-most-health-decisions-in-the-home.

15 "20 Reasons for Blood Sugar Swings," WebMD, medically reviewed November 1, 2019, https://www.webmd.com/diabetes/daily-control-19/treat/slideshow-blood-sugar-swings.

16 T. J. Wahls, "The Seventy Percent Solution," Journal General Internal Medicine 26, no. 10 (2011): 1215–16.

17 Melonie Heron, "Deaths: Leading Causes for 2017," National Vital Statistics Reports 68, no. 6 (2019).

18 "Know Your Health Numbers," American Heart Association, last reviewed August 31, 2015, https://www.heart.org/en/health-topics/diabetes/prevention--treatment-of-diabetes/know-your-health-numbers.

19 Marlene Goldman, Rebecca Troisi, and Kathryn Rexrode, Women & Health (San Diego: Academic Press, 2013), 96.

20 "Breast Exam: Breast Cancer Screenings" Johns Hopkins Medicine, accessed May 4, 2020, https://www.hopkinsmedicine.org/kimmel cancer center/centers/breast cancer program/treatment and services/risk and prevention/breast exam.html.

21 "American Cancer Society Recommendations for the Early Detection of Breast Cancer," American Cancer Society, last revised March 5, 2020, https://www.cancer.org/cancer/breast-cancer/screening-test s-and-early-detection/american-cancer-society-recommendati ons-for-the-early-detection-of-breast-cancer.html.

22 "American Cancer Society Recommendations."

23 "American Cancer Society Recommendations."

24 "American Cancer Society Recommendations."

25 "Health Screenings for Women Ages 18 to 39," MedlinePlus, accessed January 18, 2020, https://medlineplus.gov/ency/article/007462.htm.

26 "Health Screenings for Women."

27 "Health Screenings for Women."

28 "Health Screenings for Women."

29 "Health Screenings for Women."

30 "4 Important Blood Tests for Women—and What the Results Mean," *Harvard Women's Health Watch*, February 21, 2014, https://www. health.harvard.edu/staying-healthy/4-important-blood-tests-for-wo men-and-what-the-results-mean.

31 "Screening for Colorectal Cancer: US Preventive Services Task Force Recommendation," Office of Disease Prevention and Health Promotion, https://www.healthypeople.gov/2020/tools-resources/ evidence-based-resource/screening-for-colorectal-cancer-u s-preventive-services.

32 "American Cancer Society Guideline for Colorectal Cancer Screening," American Cancer Society, last revised May 30,

2018, https://www.cancer.org/cancer/colon-rectal-cancer/detection-diagnosis-staging/acs-recommendations.html.

33 David Turbert, "Eye Exam and Vision Testing Basics," American Academy of Ophthalmology, December 17, 2018, https://www.aao.org/eye-health/tips-prevention/eye-exams-101.

34 "Key Facts About Influenza (Flu)," Centers for Disease Control and Prevention, National Center for Immunization and Respiratory Diseases (NCIRD), last reviewed September 13, 2019, https://www.cdc.gov/flu/about/keyfacts.htm.

35 "Diphtheria, Tetanus, and Pertussis Vaccine Recommendations," National Center for Immunization and Respiratory Diseases, last reviewed January 22, 2020, https://www.cdc.gov/vaccines/vpd/dtap-tdap-td/hcp/recommendations.html.

36 "What is Osteoporosis?," International Osteoporosis Foundation, 2017, https://www.iofbonehealth.org/what-is-osteoporosis.

37 "Osteoporosis," Mayo Clinic on Diseases and Conditions, 2019 https://www.mayoclinic.org/diseases-conditions/osteoporosis/symptoms-causes/syc-20351968.

38 "How Osteoporosis Is Diagnosed," Mayo Clinic, accessed January 20, 2020, https://www.mayoclinic.org/diseases-conditions/osteoporosis/in-depth/osteoporosis/art-20304599.

39 "Does Osteoporosis Run in Your Family?," Centers for Disease Control and Prevention, reviewed July 5, 2019, https://www.cdc.gov/genomics/disease/osteoporosis.htm?CDC_AA_refVal=https%3A%2F%2Fwww.cdc.gov%2Ffeatures%2Fosteoporosis%2Findex.html.

40 "About Adult BMI," Division of Nutrition, Physical Activity, and Obesity; National Center for Chronic Disease Prevention and Health Promotion, last reviewed April 10, 2020. https://www.cdc.gov/healthyweight/assessing/bmi/adult_bmi/index.html.

41 "Understanding Blood Pressure Readings," American Heart Association, last reviewed November 30, 2017, https://www.heart.org/en/health-topics/high-blood-pressure/understanding-blood-pressure-readings.

42   Jenna Fletcher, "What Should My Cholesterol Level Be at My Age?," *Medical News Today*, last reviewed on January 5, 2020, https://www.medicalnewstoday.com/articles/315900.

43   Michael Dansinger, "Prediabetes (Borderline Diabetes)," WebMD, last reviewed December 13, 2019, https://www.webmd.com/diabetes/what-is-prediabetes.

44   Michael Greger, *How Not to Diet* (New York: Flatiron Books, 2019).

45   Phillip Watson, Andrew Whale, Stephen A. Mears, Louise A. Reyner, and Ronald J. Maughan, "Mild Hypohydration Increases the Frequency of Driver Errors During a Prolonged, Monotonous Driving Task," *Journal of Physiology & Behavior* 147 (August 2015): 313–18.

46   "Sugary Drinks in America: Who's Drinking What and How Much?," Health Food America, accessed January 16, 2020, http://www.healthyfoodamerica.org/sugary_drinks_in_america_who_s_drinking_what_and_how_much.

47   "How Many Cups of Coffee Do You Personally Drink on Average per Day at Home During the Week?," Statista, February 11, 2020, https://www.statista.com/statistics/250230/americans-daily-coffee-consumption/.

48   "Excessive Alcohol Use and Risks to Women's Health," Division of Population Health, National Center for Chronic Disease Prevention and Health Promotion, Centers for Disease Control and Prevention, last reviewed December 30, 2019, https://www.cdc.gov/alcohol/fact-sheets/womens-health.htm

49   "The Water in You: Water and the Human Body," USGS Science for a Changing World, accessed January 20, 2020, https://www.usgs.gov/special-topic/water-science-school/science/water-you-water-and-human-body?qt-science_center_objects=0#qt-science_center_objects.

50   "What Is Dehydration? What Causes It?," WebMD, last reviewed May 30, 2019, https://www.webmd.com/a-to-z-guides/dehydration-adults#1.

51   Gina Shaw, "Water and Your Diet: Staying Slim and Regular With H2O," WebMD, last reviewed July 7, 2009, https://www.webmd.com/diet/features/water-for-weight-loss-diet#2.

52   SC Hauser, "Recipe for Healthy Digestion," in *Mayo Clinic on Digestive Health*, 3rd ed. (Rochester, MN: Mayo Foundation for Medical Education and Research, 2011).

53   Gretchen Reynolds, "Bananas vs. Sports Drinks?," *The New York Times*, April 4, 2018.

54   "Sugary Drinks in America."

55   James McIntosh, "Fifteen Benefits of Drinking Water," *Medical News Today*, July 16, 2018, https://www.medicalnewstoday.com/articles/290814#benefits.

56   Kris Gunnars, "10 Evidence-Based Benefits of Green Tea," *Healthline*, April 6, 2020, https://www.healthline.com/nutrition/top-10-evidence-based-health-benefits-of-green-tea#1.-Contains-healthy-bio-active-compounds.

57   "Caffeine: How Much Is Too Much?," Mayo Clinic, accessed January 15, 2020, https://www.mayoclinic.org/healthy-lifestyle/nutrition-and-healthy-eating/in-depth/caffeine/art-20045678.

58   "Spilling the Beans—How Much Caffeine Is Too Much?," US Food & Drug Administration, reviewed December 12, 2018, https://www.fda.gov/consumers/consumer-updates/spilling-beans-how-much-caffeine-too-much.

59   "Women and Alcohol," National Institute on Alcohol Abuse and Alcoholism, December 2019, https://www.niaaa.nih.gov/publications/brochures-and-fact-sheets/women-and-alcohol.

60   Alice G. Walton, "People in the U.S. Are Drinking More Alcohol Than Ever: Study," *Forbes*, August 17, 2017, https://www.forbes.com/sites/alicegwalton/2017/08/12/people-in-the-u-s-are-drinking-more-alcohol-than-ever-study/#1d1678023eb7.

61   "Alcohol Use and Your Health" Division of Population Health, National Center for Chronic Disease Prevention and Health Promotion, Centers

for Disease Control and Prevention. December 30, 2019, https://www.cdc.gov/alcohol/fact-sheets/alcohol-use.htm.

62   "Alcohol Use and Your Health."

63   "Is It Safe for Women to Drink Alcohol?," *Harvard Health Letter*, November 2018, https://www.health.harvard.edu/womens-health/is-it-safe-for-women-to-drink-alcohol.

64   "Is It Safe for Women to Drink Alcohol?"

65   "Excessive Alcohol Use and Risks to Women's Health," Division of Population Health, National Center for Chronic Disease Prevention and Health Promotion, Centers for Disease Control and Prevention, last reviewed December 30, 2019, https://www.cdc.gov/alcohol/fact-sheets/womens-health.htm.

66   "Is It Safe for Women to Drink Alcohol?"

67   "How Much Sugar Is Too Much?," American Heart Association, accessed May 4, 2020, https://www.heart.org/en/healthy-living/healthy-eating/eat-smart/sugar/how-much-sugar-is-too-much.

68   "Caffeine: How Much Is Too Much?"

69   Tara Parker-Pope, "Make 2020 the Year of Less Sugar," *The New York Times*, December 30, 2019.

70   Parker-Pope, "Make 2020."

71   "Globally, One in Five Deaths Are Associated with Poor Diet," *The Lancet*, April 3, 2019, https://www.sciencedaily.com/releases/2019/04/190403193702.htm.

72   Wullianallur Raghupathi and Viju Raghupathi, "An Empirical Study of Chronic Diseases in the United States: A Visual Analytics Approach to Public Health," *International Journal of Environmental Research and Public Health* 15 (2018): 431–39.

73   Cheryl D. Fryar, Jeffery P. Hughes, Kirsten A. Herrick, and Namanjeet Ahluwalia, "Fast Food Consumption Among Adults in the United

States, 2013–2016," National Center for Health Statistics, Brief No. 322, October 2018, https://www.cdc.gov/nchs/products/databriefs/db322.htm.

74 Sara Sloat, "How Much Do Humans Eat By The Numbers?," Inverse, accessed February 3, 2010, https://www.inverse.com/article/38623-pounds-of-food-united-states-calories.

75 Amanda Capritto, "How to Calculate and Track Your Macros," CNET, updated December 2019, https://www.cnet.com/how-to/how-to-track-your-macros-guide.

76 Ashley Marcin, "How Many Calories Do I Burn in a Day?," Healthline, May 3, 2017, https://www.healthline.com/health/fitness-exercise/how-many-calories-do-i-burn-a-day.

77 A. C. Ross et al., "Dietary Reference Intakes (DRIs): Acceptable Macronutrient Distribution Ranges," The National Academies Press, 2011, https://www.ncbi.nlm.nih.gov/books/NBK56068/table/summarytables.t5/?report=objectonly.

78 "Get to Know Carbs," American Diabetes Association, accessed January 3, 2020, https://www.diabetes.org/nutrition/understanding-carbs.

79 Sanjay Sharma, "Food Preservatives and Their Harmful Effects," International Journal of Scientific and Research Publications 5, no. 4 (April 2015), http://www.ijsrp.org/research-paper-0415/ijsrp-p4014.pdf.

80 Gavin Van De Walle, "What Are Simple Sugars? Simple Carbohydrates Explained," Healthline, January 7, 2019, https://www.healthline.com/nutrition/simple-sugars.

81 Madelyn Fernstrom, "Hungry? These Foods Will Keep You Full Longer," Today, April 25, 2017, https://www.today.com/health/these-foods-will-ward-hunger-keep-you-full-t110761.

82 Fernstrom, "Hungry?"

83 "How Much Sugar Is Too Much?"

84 James M. Lattimer and Mark D. Haub, "Effects of Dietary Fiber and Its Components on Metabolic Health," *Nutrients* 2, no. 12 (December 2010): 1266–89.

85 R. Clemens et al., "Filling America's Fiber Intake Gap: Summary of a Roundtable to Probe Realistic Solutions with a Focus on Grain-Based Foods," *Journal Nutrition* 142, no. 7: 139-140.

86 Holly Larson, "Easy Ways to Boost Fiber in Your Daily Diet," Academy of Nutrition and Dietetics, December 19, 2019, https://www.eatright.org/food/vitamins-and-supplements/types-of-vitamins-and-nutrients/easy-ways-to-boost-fiber-in-your-daily-diet.

87 "Carb Counts," Centers for Disease Control and Prevention, last reviewed March 21, 2019, https://www.cdc.gov/diabetes/managing/eat-well/diabetes-and-carbs/carbohydrate-choice-lists.html.

88 "Protein—What Is It and Why Should We Care?" *Healthline*, accessed January 5, 2020, https://www.healthline.com/nutrition/how-much-protein-per-day#what-it-is.

89 "Plant-Based Diets: A Physician's Guide," *The Permanente Journal*, July 6, 2016, https://www.ncbi.nlm.nih.gov/pmc/articles/PMC4991921/.

90 "Plant-Based Diets."

91 Christopher Graffeo, "Is There Evidence to Support a Vegetarian Diet in Common Chronic Diseases?," *Clinical Correlations*, June 20, 2013, www.clinicalcorrelations.org/?p=6186.

92 Graffeo, "Is There Evidence to Support a Vegetarian Diet In Common Chronic Diseases?"

93 Heidi Lynch, Carol Johnston, and Christopher Wharton, "Plant-Based Diets: Considerations for Environmental Impact, Protein Quality, and Exercise Performance," *Nutrients*, December 10, 2018, https://www.ncbi.nlm.nih.gov/pmc/articles/PMC6316289/.

94 Kelli McGrane, "13 Nearly Complete Protein Sources for Vegetarians and Vegans," *Healthline*, April 21, 2020, https://www.healthline.com/nutrition/complete-protein-for-vegans.

95   McGrane, "13 Nearly Complete."

96   Stefan M. Pasiakos, Sanjiv Agarwal, Harris R. Lieberman, and Victor L. Fulgoni III, "Sources and Amounts of Animal, Dairy, and Plant Protein Intake of US Adults in 2007–2010," *Nutrients*, August 21, 2015, https://www.ncbi.nlm.nih.gov/pmc/articles/PMC4555161/.

97   "FAQ: Processed Meat and Cancer," American Institute for Cancer Research, August 7, 2014, https://www.aicr.org/news/faq-processed-meat-and-cancer/.

98   "Protein Content of Foods," *Today's Dietitian*, 2013, https://www.todaysdietitian.com/pdf/webinars/ProteinContentofFoods.pdf.

99   "Protein Content of Foods."

100 Jessie Szalay, "What Is Dietary Fat?," *Live Science*, December 18, 2015, https://www.livescience.com/53145-dietary-fat.html.

101 Jayne Leonard, "Understanding Healthful vs. Unhealthful Fats," *Medical News Today*, reviewed June 28, 2018, https://www.medicalnewstoday.com/articles/322295.php#understanding-healthful-vs-unhealthful-fats.

102 "Types of Fat," The Nutrition Source, Harvard T. H. Chan School of Public Health, https://www.hsph.harvard.edu/nutritionsource/what-should-you-eat/fats-and-cholesterol/types-of-fat/.

103 Jayne Leonard, "What Are the Most Healthful High-Fat Foods?" *Medical News Today*, June 28, 2018, https://www.medicalnewstoday.com/articles/322295.

104 "2015–2020 Dietary Guidelines for Americans," US Department of Health and Human Services and US Department of Agriculture, accessed February 7, 2020, http://health.gov/dietaryguidelines/2015/guidelines/.

105 Leonard, "What Are the Most Healthful High-Fat Foods?"

106 "2015–2020 Dietary Guidelines."

107 "2015–2020 Dietary Guidelines."

108 "Reading Food Labels," The Society for Cardiovascular Angiography and Interventions, August 6, 2014, http://www.secondscount.org/healthy-living/healthy-living-detail-2/reading-food-labels-2#.Xq2IyC2ZPOQ.

109 "The Truth about Fats: The Good, the Bad, and the In-Between," Harvard Health Publishing, Harvard Medical School, last updated December 11, 2019, https://www.health.harvard.edu/staying-healthy/the-truth-about-fats-bad-and-good.

110 "By the Way, Doctor: Is Palm Oil Good for You?," Harvard Health Publishing, Harvard Medical School, last updated March 18, 2019, https://www.health.harvard.edu/staying-healthy/by the way doctor is palm oil good for you.

111 K. M. Dickinson, P. M. Clifton, and J. B. Deogh, "Endothelial Function Is Impaired after a High-Salty Meal in Healthy Study Subjects," American Journal of Clinical Nutrition 93, no. 3: 500–505.

112 "2015–2020 Dietary Guidelines."

113 Greger, How Not to Diet, 574–93.

114 "Dietary Reference Intakes for Calcium and Vitamin D," National Academies of Sciences, Engineering, and Medicine, accessed December 2, 2018, https://www.nap.edu/catalog/13050/dietary-reference-intakes-for-calcium-and-vitamin-d.

115 "Increasing Calcium in Your Diet," Cleveland Clinic, January 3, 2020, https://my.clevelandclinic.org/health/drugs/16297-increasing-calcium-in-your-diet.

116 Suzanne Hinck, "When Going Organic Matters Most for You," Cleveland Clinic, July 10, 2014, https://health.clevelandclinic.org/when-going-organic-matters-most-for-you/.

117 Dagfinn Aune, Edward Giovannucci, Paolo Boffetta, Lars T. Fadnes, NaNa Keum, Teresa Norat, Darren C. Greenwood, Elio Riboli, Lars J. Vatten, and Serena Tonstad, "Fruit and Vegetable Intake and the Risk of Cardiovascular Disease, Total Cancer and All-Cause

Mortality—A Systematic Review and Dose-Response Meta-Analysis of Prospective Studies," *Oxford Journals: International Journal of Epidemiology*, June 2017, https://www.ncbi.nlm.nih.gov/pmc/articles/PMC5837313/.

118 Sarah Klemm, "Healthy Eating for Women," Academy of Nutrition and Dietetics, last reviewed April 2020, https://www.eatright.org/food/nutrition/dietary-guidelines-and-myplate/healthy-eating-for-women.

119 "Benefits of Physical Activity," Division of Nutrition, Physical Activity, and Obesity; National Center for Chronic Disease Prevention and Health Promotion, last reviewed April 10, 2020, https://www.cdc.gov/physicalactivity/basics/pa-health/index.htm.

120 "Physical Activity and Health: A Report of the Surgeon General," Centers for Disease Control and Prevention, accessed January 10, 2020, https://www.cdc.gov/nccdphp/sgr/women.htm.

121 "Physical Activity and Health."

122 "Physical Activity and Health."

123 "Why Is Physical Activity So Important for Health and Well-Being?," American Heart Association, last reviewed January 14, 2017, https://www.heart.org/en/healthy-living/fitness/fitness-basics/why-is-physical-activity-so-important-for-health-and-wellbeing.

124 US Department of Health and Human Services, *Physical Activity Guidelines for Americans*, February 1, 2019, https://www.hhs.gov/fitness/be-active/physical-activity-guidelines-for-americans/index.html.

125 Department of Health and Human Services, "Key Guidelines," in *Physical Activity Guidelines for Americans*, 2nd ed. (2018), 8, https://health.gov/sites/default/files/2019-09/Physical_Activity_Guidelines_2nd_edition.pdf.

126 Department of Health and Human Services, "Key Guidelines," 8.

127 Department of Health and Human Services, "Key Guidelines," 8.

128 Meredith L. Birsner and Cynthia Gyamfi-Bannerman, "Physical Activity and Exercise During Pregnancy and the Postpartum Period," *The American College of Obstetricians and Gynecologists*, no. 84 (April 2020), https://www.acog.org/clinical/clinical-guidance/committee-opinion/articles/2020/04/physical-activity-and-exercise-during-pregnancy-and-the-postpartum-period.

129 Erica Oberg, "Physical Activity Prescription: Our Best Medicine," *Integrative Medicine* 6, no. 5 (October/November 2007).

130 Wendy Bumgardner, "Target Heart Rate Calculator Chart," Verywell Fit, December 2, 2019, https://www.verywellfit.com/target-heart-rate-calculator-3878160.

131 "Know Your Target Heart Rates for Exercise, Losing Weight and Health," American Heart Association, accessed on November 1, 2019, https://www.heart.org/en/healthy-living/fitness/fitness-basics/target-heart-rates.

132 "Physical Activity Guidelines for Americans."

133 Laurel Leicht, "So Does Muscle Weigh More Than Fat, or What?," *Prevention*, November 6, 2018, https://www.prevention.com/fitness/workouts/a20452238/does-muscle-weigh-more-than-fat-0/.

134 "1 in 3 Adults Don't Get Enough Sleep," Centers for Disease Control and Prevention, accessed January 18, 2020, https://www.cdc.gov/media/releases/2016/p0215-enough-sleep.html.

135 Lauren Vinopal Fatherly, "Women Actually Do Need More Sleep than Men," *Business Insider,* February 21, 2017, https://www.businessinsider.com/why-women-need-more-sleep-2017-2.

136 "1 in 3 Adults."

137 "Women and Sleep," National Sleep Foundation, accessed on May 3, 2020, https://www.sleepfoundation.org/articles/women-and-sleep.

138 "How Does Sleep Affect Your Heart Health?," National Center for Chronic Disease Prevention and Health Promotion, Division for Heart Disease and Stroke Prevention, last reviewed December 3, 2018, https://www.cdc.gov/features/sleep-heart-health/index.html.

139 "Insomnia and Women," National Sleep Foundation, accessed November 3, 2019, https://www.sleepfoundation.org/insomnia/insomnia-you/insomnia-women.

140 "Sleep Disorders Affect Men and Women Differently," American Academy of Sleep Medicine, May 23, 2017, https://www.sciencedaily.com/releases/2017/05/170523081838.htm.

141 N. F. Watson, M. S. Badr, G. Belenky, D. L. Bliwise, O. M. Buxton, D. Buysse, D. F. Dinges, J. Gangwisch, M. A. Grandner, C. Kushida, R. K. Malhotra, J. L. Martin, S. R. Patel, S. F. Quan, and E. Tasali, "Recommended Amount of Sleep for a Healthy Adult: A Joint Consensus Statement of the American Academy of Sleep Medicine and Sleep Research Society," *SLEEP*, June 1, 2015, https://www.ncbi.nlm.nih.gov/pubmed/26039963.

142 "What to Do When You Can't Sleep," National Sleep Foundation, accessed on May 3, 2020, https://www.sleepfoundation.org/insomnia/treatment/what-do-when-you-cant-sleep.

143 Beverly Hosford, "When Is the Best Time of Day to Exercise?," American Council on Exercise, February 6, 2018, https://www.acefitness.org/education-and-resources/professional/expert-articles/6929/when-is-the-best-time-of-day-to-exercise/.

144 Hosford, "Best Time of Day to Exercise."

145 Kerstin Uvnäs-Moberg, Lina Handlin, and Maria Petersson, "Self-Soothing behaviors with Particular Reference to Oxytocin Release Induced by Non-Noxious Sensory Stimulation," *Frontiers in Psychology*, January 12, 2015, https://www.frontiersin.org/articles/10.3389/fpsyg.2014.01529/full.

146 "Napping," National Sleep Foundation, accessed on May 3, 2020, https://www.sleepfoundation.org/articles/napping.

147 "Results from the 2017 National Survey on Drug Use and Health," Substance Abuse and Mental Health Services Administration Center for Behavioral Health Statistics and Quality, 2018, https://www.samhsa.gov/data/sites/default/files/cbhsq-reports/NSDUHDetailedTabs2017/NSDUHDetailedTabs2017.pdf.

148 "5 Things You Should Know About Stress," The National Institute of Mental Health, NIH Publication No. 19-MH-8109, https://www.nimh.nih.gov/health/publications/stress/index.shtml.

149 "Mental Health Information: Statistics," The National Institute of Mental Health, last updated January 2018, https://www.nimh.nih.gov/health/statistics/index.shtml.

150 K. A. Yonkers and R. F. Casper, R. F., "Epidemiology and Pathogenesis of Premenstrual Syndrome and Premenstrual Dysphoric Disorder," eds. R. L. Barbieri and W. F. Crowley Jr., January 15, 2018, from https://www.uptodate.com/contents/epidemiology-and-pathogenesis-of-premenstrual-syndrome-and-premenstrual-dysphoric-disorder?topicRef=7382&source=see_link.

151 J. Y. Ko, K. M. Rockhill, V. T. Tong, B. Morrow, S. L. Farr, "Trends in Postpartum Depressive Symptoms—27 States, 2004, 2008, and 2012," *Morbidity and Mortality Weekly Report* 66 (2017): 153–58.

152 Oren Jay Sofer, "Balance: Overwhelming Emotions," interview by Dan Harris, January 22, 2020, in *Ten Percent Happier*, podcast.

153 Sofer, "Balance: Overwhelming Emotions."

154 Kate L. Brookie, Georgia I. Best, and Tamlin S. Conner, "Intake of Raw Fruits and Vegetables Is Associated with Better Mental Health Than Intake of Processed Fruits and Vegetables," *Frontiers in Psychology* 9 (2018): 487.

155 "Depression and Anxiety: Exercise Eases Symptoms," Mayo Clinic, September 27, 2017, https://www.mayoclinic.org/diseases-conditions/depression/in-depth/depression-and-exercise/art-20046495.

156 E. Kim, V. Strecher, and C. Ryff, "Purpose in Life and Use of Preventive Health Care Services," *Proceedings of the National Academy of Sciences of the United States of America* 111, no. 46: 16331–36, doi:10.1073/pnas.1414826111. https://www.ncbi.nlm.nih.gov/pmc/articles/PMC4246300.

157 P. Boyle, A. Buchman, R. Wilson, L. Yu, J. Schneider, and D. Bennett, "Effect of Purpose in Life on the Relation between Alzheimer Disease Pathologic Changes on Cognitive Function in Advanced Age," *Arch*

Gen Psychiatry 69, no. 5 (May 2012):499–505, doi: 10.1001/archgenpsychiatry.2011.1487. https://www.ncbi.nlm.nih.gov/pubmed/22566582.

158 S. Hooker and K. Masters, "Purpose in Life Is Associated with Physical Activity Measured by Accelerometer," *Journal of Health Psychology* 21 (2016): 962–71, doi.org/10.1177/1359105314542822. https://journals.sagepub.com/doi/10.1177/1359105314542822

159 Linda Wasmer Andrews, "How a Sense of Purpose in Life Improves Your Health. A More Meaningful Life Is Likely to Be Healthier as Well. Here's Why," *Minding the Body* (blog), *Psychology Today*, July 14, 2017, https://www.psychologytoday.com/us/blog/minding-the-body/201707/how-sense-purpose-in-life-improves-your-health.

160 Mount Sinai Medical Center, "Have a Sense of Purpose in Life? It May Protect Your Heart," *ScienceDaily*, www.sciencedaily.com/releases/2015/03/150306132538.htm.

161 P. Jaret, "Does Your Life Have Purpose?," Berkeley Wellness, May 23, 2016, https://www.berkeleywellness.com/healthy-mind/mind-body/article/does-your-life-have-purpose.

162 P. Hill and N. Turiano, "Purpose in Life as a Predictor of Mortality across Adulthood," *Psychological Science* 25, no. 7 (July 2014): 1482–86, doi: 10.1177/0956797614531799. https://www.ncbi.nlm.nih.gov/pmc/articles/PMC4224996.

163 P. Hill, N. Turiano, D. Mroczek, and A. Burrow, "The Value of a Purposeful Life: Sense of Purpose Predicts Greater Income and Net Worth," *Journal of Research in Personality* 65 (2016): 38–42, doi:10.1016/j.jrp.2016.07.003. https://www.ncbi.nlm.nih.gov/pmc/articles/PMC5408461.

164 J. Chochovski, G. Kennedy, and A. Anderson, "Ageing and Depression: Sense of Purpose, Self-Efficacy, Values and Self-Esteem as Protective Factors," *Journal of Aging Science*, 2016, https://www.longdom.org/proceedings/ageing-and-depression-sense-of-purpose-selfefficacy-values-and-selfesteem-as-protective-factors-7399.html.

165 A. Turner, C. Smith, and J. Ong, "Is Purpose in Life Associated with Less Sleep Disturbance in Older Adults?," *Sleep Science Practice* 1, no.

14 (2017), doi:10.1186/s41606-017-0015-6. https://sleep.biomedcentral.
com/articles/10.1186/s41606-017-0015-6#citeas.

166 G. Chapman, *The 5 Love Languages* (Chicago: Northfield Publishing, 2015).

167 T. Hartman, *The Color Code Personality Profile* (Color Code International, 2011).

168 L. Ellis and M. Anderson, *The Dash: Making a Difference with Your Life* (Naperville, IL: Simple Truths, 2005).

169 Chris Branter, "The Connection Between Sex and Sleep," *Psychology Today*, August 22, 2018, https://www.psychologyto-day.com/us/blog/the-truth-about-exercise-addiction/201808/the-connection-between-sex-and-sleep.

170 R. C. Rosen, "Prevalence and Risk Factors of Sexual Dysfunction in Men and Women," *Current Psychiatry Reports*, no. 3 (June 2000): 189–95, https://www.ncbi.nlm.nih.gov/pubmed/11122954.

171 "Female Sexual Dysfunction," WebMD, last Reviewed May 7, 2019, https://www.webmd.com/women/guide/sexual-dysfunction-women#1.

172 Bernice Yeung, "Here Are 3 Startling New Stats on Rape," *Reveal*, November 2, 2017, https://www.revealnews.org/blog/here-are-three-startling-new-stats-on-rape/.

173 J. Grohol, "11 Surprising Facts About America's Sexual Behaviors," *Psych Central*, accessed January 22, 2020, https://psychcentral.com/blog/11-surprising-facts-about-americas-sexual-behaviors.

174 J. M. Twenge, R. A. Sherman, and B. E. Wells, "Declines in Sexual Frequency among American Adults, 1989–2014," *Archives of Sexual Behavior* 46 (2017): 2389–401, https://doi.org/10.1007/s10508-017-0953-1.

175 Twenge, Sherman, and Wells, "Declines in Sexual Frequency."

176 Jessie V. Ford, Rheta Barnes, Anne Rompalo, and Edward W. Hook III, "Sexual Health Training and Education in the U.S.," supplement, *Public Health Reports* 128, no. S1 (March–April 2013): 96–101, https://www.ncbi.nlm.nih.gov/pmc/articles/PMC3562751/.

177 "Menstrual Cycle," US Department of Health and Human Services: Office on Women's Health, last updated April 25, 2018, https://www.womenshealth.gov/menstrual-cycle.

178 "Menstrual Cycle: What's Normal, What's Not," Mayo Clinic, June 13, 2019, https://www.mayoclinic.org/healthy-lifestyle/womens-health/in-depth/menstrual-cycle/art-20047186.

179 K. E. Barrett et al., "Reproductive Development & Function of the Female Reproductive System," in *Ganong's Review of Medical Physiology*, 26th ed. (New York: McGraw-Hill Education, 2019).

180 Charles Patrick Davis, "What Should I Know about Menstruation (Monthly Period)? What Is the Medical Definition of It?," MedicineNet, accessed May 4, 2020, https://www.medicinenet.com/menstruation/article.htm.

181 Michael Castleman, "The Most Important Sexual Statistic— Intercourse Is Not the Key to Most Women's Sexual Satisfaction," *Psychology Today*, March 16, 2009.

182 Len Canter, "Douching: More Harmful Than Helpful," *U.S. News & World Report*, April 2, 2019, https://www.usnews.com/news/health-news/articles/2019-04-02/douching-more-harmful-than-helpful.

183 Rosemary Basson, "Overview of Sexual Dysfunction in Women," Merck Manual, last modified February 2014, https://www.merckmanuals.com/home/women-s-health-issues/sexual-dysfunction-in-women/overview-of-sexual-dysfunction-in-women.

184 Sheryl A. Kingsberg, "Attitudinal Survey of Women Living with Low Sexual Desire," *Journal of Women's Health* 23, no. 10 (2014).

185 Kingsberg, "Attitudinal Survey of Women."

186 Kingsberg, "Genitourinary Syndrome of Menopause: New Terminology for Vulvovaginal Atrophy from the International Society

for the Study of Women's Sexual Health and the North American Menopause Society," *Menopause: The Journal of the North American Menopause Society* 21, no. 10: 1063–68.

187 Kingsberg, "Genitourinary Syndrome of Menopause," 1063–68.

188 Kingsberg, "Genitourinary Syndrome of Menopause," 1063–68.

189 Holly N. Thomas and Rebecca C. Thurston, "A Biopsychosocial Approach to Women's Sexual Function and Dysfunction at Midlife: A Narrative Review," *Maturitas*, February 21, 2016, doi: 10.1016/j.maturitas.2016.02.009.

190 Thomas and Thurston, "A Biopsychosocial Approach."

191 Thomas and Thurston, "A Biopsychosocial Approach."

192 Thomas and Thurston, "A Biopsychosocial Approach."

193 Reece D. Herbenick, M. Reece, S. Sander, B. Dodge, A. Ghassemi, and J. D. Fortenberry, "Prevalence and Characteristics of Vibrator Use by Women in the United States: Results from a Nationally Representative Study," *Journal of Sex Medicine* 6, no. 7 (July 2009): 1857–66, doi: 10.1111/j.1743-6109.2009.01318.x.

194 J. R. Cates, N. L. Herndon, S. L. Schulz, J. E. Darroch, "Our Voices, Our Lives, Our Futures: Youth and Sexually Transmitted Diseases," (Chapel Hill, NC: University of North Carolina at Chapel Hill School of Journalism and Mass Communication, 2004).

195 "Sexually Transmitted Diseases," Office of Disease Prevention and Health promotion, accessed May 4, 2020, https://www.healthypeople.gov/2020/topics-objectives/topic/sexually-transmitted-diseases.

196 H. W. Chesson, E. F. Dunne, S. Hariri, and L. E. Markowitz, "The Estimated Lifetime Probability of Acquiring Human Papillomavirus in the United States," *Sexually Transmitted Diseases*. 41, no. 11 (November 2014): 660–64.

197 G. McQuillan, D. Kruszon-Moran, E. W. Flagg, and R. Paulose-Ram, "Prevalence of Herpes Simplex Virus Type 1 and Type 2 in Persons

Aged 14–49: United States, 2015–2016," NCHS Data Brief, no. 304 (Hyattsville, MD: National Center for Health Statistics, 2018).

198 "Safe Sex for Older Adults," HealthinAging.org, last updated August 2019, https://www.healthinaging.org/tools-and-tips/safe-sex-older-adults.

199 Melissa Conrad Stöppler, "Menopause," MedicineNet, accessed on May 4, 2020, https://www.medicinenet.com/menopause/article.htm.

200 Stöppler, "Menopause."

201 Sonam Sheth, Shayanne Gal, and Madison Hoff, "7 Charts That Show the Glaring Gap between Men's and Women's Salaries in the U.S.," Business Insider, March 31, 2020, https://www.businessinsider.com/gender-wage-pay-gap-charts-2017-3

202 Jennifer Erin Brown, "New Research Finds 95 Percent of Millennials Not Saving Adequately for Retirement," February 27, 2018, https://www.nirsonline.org/2018/02/new-research-finds-95-percent-of-millennials-not-saving-adequately-for-retirement/.

203 Zhe Li and Joseph Dalaker, "Poverty Among Americans Aged 65 and Older," Congressional Research Service, R45791, July 1, 2019, https://fas.org/sgp/crs/misc/R45791.pdf.

204 Brett Whysel, "3 Vicious Cycles: Links Among Financial, Physical And Mental Health," Forbes, June 27, 2018, https://www.forbes.com/sites/brettwhysel/2018/06/27/3-vicious-cycles/#31f0bd97540d.

205 Sarah Zeff Gerber, "Women Retiring Solo," Retirement Options, January 27, 2020, https://www.retirementoptions.com/women-retiring-solo/.

206 Neale Godfrey, "Student Loan Debt Is the Gift That Keeps Giving," Forbes, December 19, 2017, https://www.forbes.com/sites/nealegodfrey/2017/12/19/student-loan-debt/#371f0143459b.

207 Joe Resendiz, "Average Credit Card Debt in America: April 2020," ValuePenguin.com, accessed on May 4, 2020, https://www.valuepenguin.com/average-credit-card-debt#key-findings.

208 "Learn about Social Security Programs," Social Security Administration, accessed May 4, 2020, https://www.ssa.gov/planners/retire/r&m6.html.

209 Whysel, "3 Vicious Cycles."

210 "Tax Benefits for Education," Internal Revenue Service Publication 970, accessed January 22, 2020, https://www.irs.gov/pub/irs-pdf/p970.pdf.

Acknowledgments

I would like to thank my best friend, true love, and husband, Vlad. Thank you for always supporting what is important to me with your love and reassurances. I love you more than any words can ever express.

To Brandon and Jessica Agranovich, thank you for fueling me with motivation to continue to write this workbook. Your tough questions, detailed discussions regarding content, insights about targeting my audience, illustrative guidance and honest ongoing feedback have greatly impacted the evolution of this book. Thank you for being interested in this project and pushing me out of my comfort zone. I love you both.

To David Agranovich, thank you for being my role model for writing! You amaze me with your ability to artfully articulate your thoughts, always with passion and feeling. I appreciate the time you took to provide me with writer's coaching sessions. I love you.

To Cherie Lollis, I am eternally grateful to you, my wonderful sister. As we grew up together, you stepped in to fill the shoes of both a Mom and Dad for me. Cherie always encouraged me to do well in school and to work hard to get through college. Even though there was no parental love in our home, Cherie made me feel important and loved; her encouragement clearly grounded me early on. Cherie, I am so happy to have you as my sister.

Having women role models as teachers during our lifetimes can be very helpful. To Perky Grissom, my stepmom, you are my favorite role model. Perky is ninety-six years old and can run circles around most people in their twenties. Although I only got to know Perky in my adult years, I truly cherish our relationship and the love you show to our entire family. Perky has her college degree, takes care of her health, has passion for life, and is one of the most positive women I have ever met. Perky exemplifies resilience.

To Vivian Kist, my dear friend and my "adopted sister," wow, it is hard to believe this book is finally done! Thank you so much for providing your detailed expertise for the passion section of this publication. Your insight, love, support, ongoing encouragement, discussions, and interjections of humor made this writing process both tolerable and fun. There were so many days I was ready to stop, and your comforting words made me march on. I appreciated the time you spent and your honest feedback when you reviewed the entire content and your suggestion to "add pictures" to make it more entertaining to read. Thank you for your friendship and love for the past twenty-five-plus years. I'm so happy to have you in my life.

During the creation process of this workbook, I met so many wonderful women. One was MC. Thank you, MC, for taking your time to review, edit, and provide valuable feedback. You gave up your time to help me with this project and provided helpful insights to create something valuable for our target audience! Getting to know you was the best part of our journey together, and I hope we stay in touch for many years ahead.

There is a lot of information in this book and in order to help you better digest the material, I wanted to add illustrations. Each illustration has a lot of thought behind it; if you have time, go back and truly look at the images and notice that they represent all women—different shapes, sizes, and cultures. I was so pleased to find Maja Milojevic, an extremely talented artist who created all the illustrations. After spending weeks together on this part of the book, not only do we have amazing images that represent the thoughts I was hoping to convey, but I also have a new friend for life. Maja, thank you for your support, creativity, passion and the love you put into the creation of our images.

Special thanks to Kate Anderson, my longtime friend and an expert dietitian who volunteered her expertise to help me round out my nutritional ideas and guidance. Thank you, Kate, for taking your time to answer all my questions and review my nutrition content!

Mindfulness is key for total well-being. For the past thirty years, I have followed, learned about, and utilized products from Belleruth Naparstek's Health Journeys. The company offers guided experiences by foremost experts in the mind-body field that address specific health and mental health conditions as well as ones that help people relax, de-stress, and sleep better. I am grateful for the resources that Belleruth and her team provided to help the readers of this workbook as they work to improve their mental well-being.

Adding the sexual health section was important to me because I really wanted to provide some clear-cut guidance for women to better understand this area of their lives. Dr. Sheryl Kingsberg was the expert I asked for help on this section of the workbook. Dr. Kingsberg is the chief of the Division of Behavioral Medicine at MacDonald Women's Hospital/University Hospitals Cleveland Medical Center and professor of Reproductive Biology and Psychiatry at Case Western Reserve University. Her areas of clinical specialization include sexual medicine, female sexual disorders, menopause, pregnancy, postpartum mood disorders, and psychological aspects of infertility.

The financial section would not have been possible without the input from "M" Monroe. "M" provided great insight and made sure that the content included would be a great stepping-stone for women of all ages in their financial planning. Thank you for your time, passion, and care to help me with this section of the book.

Because this is a health guide, it is imperative that I provided references for any facts that were shared. As you may have noticed, there are over two hundred references. Thank you to Matt Schaffer for taking the time to work with me on the correctly formatted bibliography. Matt, I have always enjoyed working with you on all projects, but this one was very important and your help was much appreciated.

During the early process of planning and creating this guide, I was able to tap into my WellCorp team of consultants. Special thanks to Samantha Monaco for sharing your expertise in fitness, Amanda Oswald for assisting with research and input on better sleep, and Denise Rondini for your assistance on our very first draft! Special thanks to Rachel Edelman for spending time editing and providing helpful and positive feedback.

Writing this book has been a learning process for me. Thank you to Simon & Schuster/Archway Publishing for their continued guidance and support throughout this process.

Of course with any project, legal guidance was necessary. Special thanks to Kristen Hoover and Hugh Berkson from McCarthy, Lebit, Crystal & Liffman Co., LPA. Your guidance and support were helpful in directing me to this final product.

The 3 Ring Circus Team has been instrumental in helping me to create my brand and polishing my speaking skills. Thank you to Josh Linkner, Jordan Broad, Matt Ciccone and Connor Trombley. Your support has been very helpful.

As mentioned earlier during my educational journey, I attended a few colleges. Thank you to Northeast Ohio Medical University, Cleveland State University, University of Detroit Mercy and Miami Dade Community College. My education has provided me with enough knowledge to understand the importance of lifelong learning.

During my time at WellCorp I have had the pleasure of meeting some very special people. Mark Bednar is one of my teammates who I hold in very high regard. Our coworking relationship grew to something more important that has lasted a lifetime - our friendship. Mark, thank you for all the years of sharing your expertise, compassion, guidance and coaching. Having you be the final proofer for this project means a lot to me because I know it was done right and was also done from a place of love. Thank you very much.

To Deb G., Iris E., Kris W., Melissa S., Shubhada P., Swati S., and Susan T., nobody understands why we meet special people in this life's journey. We are not related by blood; we didn't know each other from the start. But God put us together to be wonderful friends by heart. Thank you for sharing so many life memories with me.

Finally, I want to make sure that I say thank you to my extended family/friends that have supported me during this lengthy process; each of these women are amazing in their own way and bring positive energy to my life and our world (listed in alphabetical order): Amalia N., Andrea G., Barbara P., Betty. B., Bella Z., Bertha C., Cheryl B., Cindy G., Diana G., Darci M., Darla H., Deb O., Enid R., Erica N., Esther B.,

Eva L., Gail N., Gail Z., Halyna P., Jackie B., Jackie W., Jane D., Jelanna O., Jill D., Johanna P., Judy H., Julie P., Julie W., Karen W., KDS, Kim Z., Lana B., Lana D., Lori L., Lisa O., Marilyn B., Marina D., Mary T., Michelle M., Rena M., Ronna N., Rosie W., Sally W., Sam L., Sharon B., Sharon H., Tammy M., Tanja L., Trisha B., Yvette W., and Zhennya B. Thank you all for your love and sisterhood.

About the Author

Cheryl Agranovich, RN, BSN, MPH

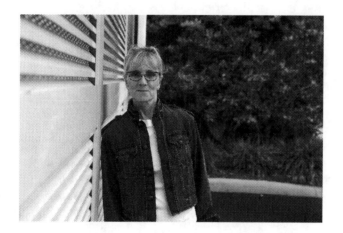

*C*heryl Agranovich was pretty much on her own during her childhood and financially independent since the age of seventeen. She was the first person in her family to go to college, and she worked full-time as she completed her degrees: registered nurse with her bachelor's in nursing and master's in public health.

She launched her health-care journey working in an emergency room, yet her interest quickly shifted to preventive health care and her career path followed. As an entrepreneur passionate about health and well-being, she founded two health companies that have helped thousands of people improve their health. Both companies were successfully sold.

Her innovative out-of-the-box thinking provided solutions to assist large multisite corporate employers, effectively enhancing their overall health and well-being strategy. Her clients included companies such as ABB, Bristol Myers Squibb, Campbell's Soup Company, Eaton, HARMAN International, IKEA, Mars, Nestle, Progressive, Scholastic Books, Sherwin Williams, and TEVA.

Cheryl shares her expertise by presenting on a national level; she addresses health and well-being topics with a targeted focus on women's health issues. She is a passionate proponent of volunteerism, supporting many important causes.

All of Cheryl's life experiences up to this point have strengthened her resolve that we can—and must—do better for our health. For that reason, she is now focusing on philanthropic efforts in health care full-time by traveling the country and giving health talks. Cheryl will use the proceeds from her speaking engagements and book sales to help young women in need succeed by funding scholarships to help them get their formal health education as well as supporting other women's health issues.